Phonobuilding

*Using Narratives
to Facilitate
Phonological
Development*

Jerry Vicino

Illustrated by Linda Wenger

*Thinking Publications
Eau Claire, Wisconsin*

00 99 98 97 96 95 94 93   8 7 6 5 4 3 2 1

Library of Congress Cataloging-in-Publication Data

Vicino, Jerry
   Phonobuilding : using narratives to facilitate phonological development / Jerry Vicino ; illustrated by Linda Wenger.
      p. cm.
  Includes bibliographical references.
  ISBN 0-930599-80-2
     1. Articulation disorders in children—Treatment. 2. Language disorders in children—Treatment. 3. Picture-writing—Therapeutic use. 4. Storytelling—Therapeutic use. I. Wenger, Linda S. II. Title.
RJ496.S7V515 1993
618.92'855—dc20
                                     92-37172
                                          CIP

Credit: The narrative examples on pages 257–259 are adapted from *Topics in Language Disorders*, Vol. 7:1, pp. 62–64, with permission from Aspen Publishers, Inc., © December 1986.

Printed in the United States of America

Thinking Publications®
A Division of McKinley Companies, Inc.

P.O. Box 163
Eau Claire, WI 54702-0163
715-832-2488
FAX: 715-832-9082

Dedication

To Doug and Camille
JLV

To my father, Albert C. Haisch,
With many loving memories
LW

Table of Contents

Overview of *Phonobuilding* 1

   Introduction 1

   Intended Population..2

   Goals of *Phonobuilding*...2

   Phonological Terms Defined 2

   Comparison of Traditional and Phonological Approaches 3

   The Influence of Hodson and Paden...4

   Phonobuilding Supports a Whole Language Philosophy 5

   Use of Pictographs 6

Phonological Approach to Remediation 7

   A Historical Perspective..7

   A Closer Look at the Phonological Approach 8

   Phonological Assessment 9

   Remediation Guidelines...10

   Phonological Cycles Approach 14

How to Use *Phonobuilding* 16

   General Procedures...16

   Monitoring Progress 19

   Using *Phonobuilding* to Develop Communication Skills 20

   Tips for Implementing *Phonobuilding*...24

   Phonobuilding Stories...25

List of Stories 27

   The Keyhole Adventure...29

   The Witch's Ride 41

   Min and the Men on the Moon 51

   The Pup Paints..63

   Nuts About Nuts...73

   Oak Tree Listens 83

   Soup Thieves...93

   Help for Mike 103

Cookies for the King 111

Come Follow Me 121

Two Ants Travel 131

Necktie Finds a New Home 141

Spoon and the Funny Spice 153

Wishing on a Star 161

Skip Dreams..169

Pups' Vacation Planning 177

Playmates for Lynn 187

Santa Saves the Sleeping Baby 197

A Rest for Rattlesnake 207

Fox and the Fat Fish 219

Sam's Magnificent Scene...227

Fox Goes to First Grade..239

Appendix A: Vocabulary Sheets..255

Appendix B: Levels of Narrative Development..................................257

References 261

Acknowledgments

Thank you to everyone who supported this project. A special thanks to Linda Schwartz-Schreiber who gave very good advice. Appreciation is also expressed to reviewers of *Phonobuilding* who graciously gave of their time to offer suggestions and improvements. A heartfelt thank you to Dr. Barbara Hodson who generously contributed her ideas and expertise. Her insightful suggestions are gratefully acknowledged. Many thanks to our wonderful families for all their helpful advice and support.

Overview of *Phonobuilding*

Introduction

Phonobuilding: Using Narratives to Facilitate Phonological Development is a holistic approach to speech and language development that uses narratives and pictographs to facilitate development of children's phonological skills. *Phonobuilding* is based on the phonological approach to remediation of speech sound disorders and is strongly influenced by the work of Hodson (1980, 1985, 1986) and Hodson and Paden (1991). Phonology is the speech sound system of a language (Hodson and Paden, 1991); a phonological approach to remediation capitalizes on the consistency of a child's phonological errors.

Pictographs—pictures that children can easily recognize—are integral to this resource. They are used to engage children ages 3 to 9 years in whole-language-based activities. Pictographs and rebus symbols, the standardized form of pictographs, have been used successfully to teach reading to English-as-a-second-language speakers, remedial readers, and other children challenged with disabilities (Bangs, 1982). Pictographs are used in *Phonobuilding* to facilitate development of children's phonological systems and communication skills.

Phonobuilding includes 22 stories, each of which is preceded by reproducible illustrations of the pictographs in the story. Pictographs replace words within the context of each story in this resource. The pictographs in each story contain one phonological pattern as defined by Hodson and Paden (1991). Each story has 10 pictographs featured within it.

The speech-language clinician reads through a chosen story with the child and allows the child to hear the spoken name of each pictograph. Target words (those represented by pictographs) have been chosen carefully to provide a facilitative phonetic context (Kent, 1982) for correct production of the target phoneme.

Children with phonological delays need to hear their target phonological patterns repeated many times (Hodson and Paden, 1991). The story format of *Phonobuilding* allows for repetition within a naturalistic context where the focus is on the meaning of the story. Children with language delays also benefit from being exposed to real stories (Goodman, Goodman, and Bird, 1991). Many children with language disorders also experience reading problems (Schory, 1990); they can quickly and easily read the pictographs in the *Phonobuilding* stories. Comprehension of *Phonobuilding* stories can be further enhanced with questioning techniques (Merritt, 1989; Schory, 1990).

Phonobuilding is based on a whole language philosophy which allows the professional to address a number of communication skills while using the pictographic stories. Phonological remediation within a narrative context enhances a child's receptive and expressive language skills, which may also be areas of weakness for the child with phonological delays (Ruscello, 1991). *Phonobuilding*

1

can be used to enhance vocabulary development, word retrieval, reasoning, question comprehension, emergent literacy skills, story retelling, and written language skills.

Phonobuilding includes a detailed description of how to use the stories to remediate phonological disorders as well as to build communication skills. A list of the stories, along with the specific pattern that each addresses, is included on pages 27–28.

Intended Population

Phonobuilding is intended for use with children between the ages of 3 and 9 who have mild to severe phonological delays (i.e., those who are mildly to severely unintelligible). Children with profound unintelligibility will need to become stimulable on target sounds before *Phonobuilding* activities will be beneficial to them. Children with language disorders and learning disabilities will also benefit from *Phonobuilding*, and it may be appropriate for children in regular education and special education programs.

The program can be used effectively for individual children or groups of children. The pictographs and the print in the stories are large enough for three or four students to see at one time. *Phonobuilding* could also be used with a large group, such as a class of students, with the distribution of multiple copies.

Goals of *Phonobuilding*

Phonobuilding can be used to:

1. develop specific phonological patterns for use in a natural environment.
2. expand vocabulary knowledge.
3. improve word-retrieval skills through the use of specific strategies.
4. enhance reasoning skills.
5. develop question comprehension.
6. develop emergent literacy skills, including holding a book appropriately, following left-to-right and front-to-back progression, and promoting understanding of the concept of a "word."
7. improve narrative skills through story retelling.
8. enhance written language skills by creating stories using pictographs.

Phonological Terms Defined

The most important terms used in describing a phonological approach to remediation and examples of each follow:

2

phonological process—is used concurrently with the terms *phonological rule* and *phonological deviation*. Currently, there is debate over which of the terms to use (Fey, 1992; Hodson, 1992a). A *phonological process* is a systematic pattern that occurs in a person's speech. In children, a phonological process often simplifies an adult phonological pattern. For example, if a child says "top" for *stop*, the phonological process being used is consonant sequence reduction. If a child says "tome" for *come*, the phonological process being used is velar fronting. A phonological process becomes *deviant* when it persists beyond a certain level and requires remediation. The identification of the phonological processes used by a child gives a description of that child's speech.

phonological pattern—is an accepted grouping within an oral language of specific sound classes, syllable shapes, and consonant sequences. For example, the phonological pattern for /sp/ is /s/ clusters, encompassing stridency and consonant sequences, and that for /k/ and /g/ is velars.

target pattern—is the adult sound class, syllable shape, or sound sequence that the child needs to acquire and that is chosen for remediation. For example, if the child uses "top" for *stop*, the target pattern would be /s/ clusters encompassing consonant sequences.

auditory stimulation—is provided when the child listens to numerous repetitions of words containing the target phoneme or pattern with low levels of amplification (Hodson and Paden, 1991).

Comparison of Traditional and Phonological Approaches

One of the major concepts separating the traditional approach to remediating speech sound disorders from the phonological approach is the remediation targets. In traditional remediation, the speech-language clinician works with the child on a specific sound. The sound is first produced by the child in isolation, then in various positions within words, words in phrases, words in sentences, etc. The child does not move to the next step in the hierarchy until reaching an accuracy rate of 80 to 90 percent.

If a child has more than one sound in error, the earliest developing or most stimulable sound (i.e., one that it is easiest for the child to produce) is addressed first. One sound is addressed until it is generally correct in conversational speech, and then the next sound is addressed. Auditory discrimination is sometimes incorporated; the child must perceive the target sound as being different from the sound he or she produces.

This is very different from phonological remediation, where specific patterns of speech are targeted. Misarticulations that a traditional approach to phonological disorders might consider random would be viewed as rule-based patterns by phonological theory. In a phonological approach, the auditory component might be stressed at the beginning and end of each session. Auditory

3

stimulation, which refers to allowing the child to hear words containing the target phoneme (usually with amplification), is a key component of the model created by Hodson and Paden (1991). (See pages 14–15 for a more thorough explanation of Hodson and Paden's phonological approach to remediation.)

The basic differences and similarities between a phonological approach and a traditional approach to phonological remediation are summarized in Table 1.1.

Table 1.1.

Phonological Approach	Traditional Approach
1. Focuses on the rules underlying the child's inaccurate productions	1. Focuses on individual error sounds
2. Targets patterns over sounds	2. Addresses one specific sound at a time
3. Can address more than one sound at a time	3. Addresses sounds singly until mastered
4. Designed for children with moderate to severe/profound unintelligibility	4. Works best for children who have mild misarticulations

Both Approaches

- Have an overall goal of helping children produce correct sounds as defined by adult speakers
- Advocate using a variety of methods to help children produce a specific sound including visual models, tactile or kinesthetic cues, and verbal directives

While *Phonobuilding* is based on a phonological approach to remediation, the stories can easily be used in traditionally based remediation. If using a traditional approach, the speech-language clinician would choose stories based on the target sound rather than the target pattern.

The Influence of Hodson and Paden

Hodson and Paden's (1991) method of phonological remediation is emphasized throughout *Phonobuilding*. Unlike other phonological approaches, theirs includes a procedure for analyzing children's error patterns as well as guidelines for remediation. Their approach is familiar to many speech-language clinicians and is structured so that assessment information from *The Assessment of Phonological Processes—Revised* (Hodson, 1986) can be used to provide a direction for remediation using *Targeting Intelligible Speech—Second Edition* (Hodson and Paden, 1991). Additionally, Hodson and Paden's approach provides that:

1. treatment of the phonological disorder is a major component of phonological remediation;

2. remediation is set up in a step-by-step fashion;
3. drill on specific patterns until a specific proficiency is attained is not advocated or recommended;
4. modifications for any clinical setting can be made; and
5. the child is actively involved in the remediation process.

Phonobuilding Supports a Whole Language Philosophy

A whole language philosophy combines the use of speaking, listening, reading, and writing skills. Specific concepts are taught within a naturalistic environment so children are engaged in meaningful experiences (Westby, 1990). Combining the skills of listening, speaking, reading, and writing aids in the development of all of them. These skills develop concurrently, not sequentially (Schory, 1990). The child is better able to integrate these skills when they are presented as related units that develop from meaningful experiences. For example, if the concept of time is being taught, the story *The Grouchy Ladybug* by Eric Carle (1977) could be used because it emphasizes time concepts.

Norris (1992) describes whole language as a principle, not a teaching method or strategy. Teaching children to read through reading and writing is one of the hallmarks of the whole language approach (Goodman, Goodman, and Bird, 1991). One of the ways this is done is by using stories that repeat many of their words or phrases, such as *Rain Makes Applesauce* by Julian Scheer (1964), or by using rhyming words such as those used in Ludwig Bemelman's *Madeline* (1939) and others in this series.

Goodman, in his book *What's Whole in Whole Language?* (1986), describes seven principles of whole language:

1. Readers construct meaning during reading.
2. Readers predict, select, confirm, and self-correct as they seek to make sense of print.
3. Writers include enough information and detail so that what they write will be comprehensible to their readers.
4. Three language systems interact in written language: the graphophonic (sound and letter patterns), the syntactic (sentence patterns), and the semantic (meanings).
5. Comprehension of meaning is always the goal of readers.
6. Expression of meaning is always what writers are trying to achieve.
7. Writers and readers are strongly limited by what they already know—writers in composing, readers in comprehending.

Addressing children's language impairments within a whole language context promotes their development of more complex oral language (Westby, 1990).

5

In *Phonobuilding*, the speech-language clinician or educator serves as a facilitator directing language activities so that children are learning and discovering listening, reading, writing, and speaking within the context of listening to, reading, writing, or discussing stories.

Using Phonobuilding *Holistically*

Using *Phonobuilding* to enhance language skills requires that the stories be examined holistically. Reading through an entire story first is very important (Schory, 1990). It is suggested that as the stories are described and discussed, the speech-language clinician should respond to the meaning of the children's responses instead of the form that the answers takes (Goodman, 1986). It is important to note that these stories do not fall under the category of "good literature" as defined by Goodman (1986) because of their contrived nature (i.e., each story needs to have a specific number of words with a specific phonological pattern/phoneme). The important skills of reading, writing, listening, and speaking, however, can still be addressed using the *Phonobuilding* narratives.

Enlarging and separating the pictographs preceding each story and allowing these to be previewed before the story is read would allow the children to create their own stories orally or in a written context. Vocabulary would then be discussed within a context-rich environment. Using themes that are present in the classroom allows for these stories to have a functional basis (Goodman et al., 1991). For example, use the *Spoon and the Funny Spice* story when talking about outerspace, or use the *Fox and the Fat Fish* story when the theme is animals and what they eat.

Phonobuilding *in the Classroom*

Integral to whole language activities is involving children in them and using the activities in a functional and purposeful manner (Goodman, 1986). An important aspect of successful use is to have the chosen *Phonobuilding* story available to the child or children in the classroom. A child who receives small-group instruction could share the pictographic story with the rest of the class by explaining and demonstrating the use of the pictographs and retelling the story. This would be an excellent language experience, because the language would be meaningful (Goodman et al., 1991). Key to the use of stories as a whole language-based activity is integration with classroom or meaningful contexts to which the child can relate (Norris and Damico, 1990).

Use of Pictographs

Pictographs are concrete pictures that closely resemble their target words (Bangs, 1982). They are often used alone, as on road signs, or in printed material to replace a printed word. They are used in texts for beginning readers and also appear in children's magazines and literature.

Pictographs have been used as an initial step in some reading programs to help children learn to read (Clark, 1974). This approach has been used successfully with children who are having difficulty learning letters and their sounds.

In a study of first and second graders' processing styles, Weed (1982) found that using visual imagery of cartoons to help children remember sentences had a positive impact on their learning of the sentences. In another study by Clark (1974), kindergarten subjects given rebus symbols learned reading material more quickly and retained the material over a longer period of time than subjects given words only.

To date, pictographs have been used as a novelty and as an aid for children who are having difficulty learning to read (Ledger and Ryan, 1982). Children with limited reading vocabulary can read more complex ideas with pictographs. They have also been widely used for communication boards. Pictographs are used in *Phonobuilding* to take advantage of visual imagery as a processing style. The children are given a visual image to match the auditory input. This gives children a visual representation for the sounds they are trying to produce.

The primary purpose of pictographs within the narratives is to offer numerous opportunities for production of the target phoneme. A single pictograph is used to represent words with multiple meanings. For instance, the pictograph for "block" is an illustration of a child's toy "block." This illustration is used to represent "block" in the context of a "city block" and "block" in the context of "preventing entry." The single pictorial representation of the multiple word meanings is less taxing for younger children to remember. For children who are capable of understanding the multiple meanings of words, however, it behooves the professional to discuss the multiple meanings of the word and to describe illustrations that might have been drawn as alternatives.

Phonological Approach to Remediation

A Historical Perspective

Phonological theory, or the idea that children's sound errors form a pattern, has been a key component in analyzing the speech of children who are unintelligible. The analysis or awareness of phonological processes that affect sound production is not new. Jakobson (1968 [1941]) first proposed the theory of phonological development by describing an orderly progression of sound development that was consistent across languages. Other theorists contributed to phonological theory with various accounts of children's phonological development, including Chomsky and Halle's (1968) Distinctive Feature Theory, Stampe's (1969) Theory of Natural Phonology, and Weiner's (1979) Minimal Pair Contrast Approach.

The work of many phonologists (Hodson, 1985, 1986; Hodson and Paden, 1991; Ingram, 1981; Khan, 1982, 1985; Khan and Lewis, 1986; Shriberg and Kwiatkowski, 1980) continues to contribute to our knowledge of phonological theory by providing frameworks for assessment of phonological processes and/or approaches to remediation. The work of these researchers and practitioners has caused speech-language clinicians to readjust their thinking and their approaches to assessing and remediating children's speech sound systems.

A Closer Look at the Phonological Approach

A phonological approach, which is used with children whose speech is severely to profoundly unintelligible, remediates broad patterns of speech rather than individual speech sounds (Weiner, 1978). The child's patterns of speech are viewed as being rule-based. When phonological processes (the broad error patterns) are identified, they can be targeted in a systematic way.

After Stampe (1969) published his Theory of Natural Phonology that described natural simplification processes, it became apparent that using this knowledge of phonological processes could help children to improve their speech in a way that was more effective than the sound-by-sound approach of traditional articulation remediation.

The advantage of a phonological approach is that focusing on the child's rule-based phonological system facilitates more rapid generalizations. For example, if a child is using the phonological process of postvocalic singleton consonant deletion, so that the word *tap* is produced as "ta" and *pat* is produced as "pa," working on the /t/ or /p/ sounds would not be productive because /t/ and /p/ are already being produced. However, working on the target pattern of word-final consonants using words with final consonant phonemes such as /t/ and /p/ would facilitate the development of word endings.

Some of the phonological treatment methods include an auditory component. This may be in the form of auditory stimulation (Hodson and Paden, 1991) or minimal pair contrasts (Weiner, 1979). The auditory or perceptual aspect of sounds is emphasized because phonological systems are believed to have two parts: underlying representations (i.e., how the child perceives the sound) and surface forms (i.e., how the child produces the sound). These two components are rule-based but are not always at the same level in a particular child. Either the sound perception or the sound production may be at a higher level (McGregor and Schwartz, 1992). Both aspects need to be addressed consistently throughout remediation.

The method of using phonological remediation to treat children with speech intelligibility problems has proven to yield quicker results with faster generalization than traditional approaches, which address one sound until mastery in conversation is achieved (Weiner, 1978). Speech-language pathologists have adopted the method of using phonological patterns to improve speech intelligibility because it has been found to be the most successful in terms of establishing intelligibility in a shorter period of time (Weiner, 1978).

Phonological Assessment

Since Stampe (1969) first described the natural processes that children use to modify their speech, a number of phonological process analysis procedures have been developed. Among the most common are these, in order of inception:

- F. Weiner's *Phonological Process Analysis* (1979);
- L. Shriberg and J. Kwiatkowski's *Natural Process Analysis* (1980);
- D. Ingram's *Procedures for the Phonological Analysis of Children's Language* (1981);
- B. Hodson's *The Assessment of Phonological Processes–Revised* (1986); and
- L. Khan and N. Lewis's *Khan-Lewis Phonological Analysis* (1986).

According to Hodson and Paden (1991), the full range of possible phonological processes children might use will never be fully cataloged. However, for a description of phonological processes most often observed in children's utterences, the reader is referred to Hodson and Paden's *Targeting Intelligible Speech—Second Edition* (1991).

Garn-Nunn and Martin (1992) studied the importance of using phonological assessment information to identify specific phonological processes in children with unintelligible speech. The diagnostic implications of looking at individual phonemes (i.e., sounds) rather than phonological processes were made clear in this study of 20 children with phonological impairments. The results of *The Assessment of Phonological Processes–Revised* (Hodson, 1986), the *Goldman-Fristoe Test of Articulation* (Goldman and Fristoe, 1986), the *Photo Articulation Test* (Pendergast, Dickey, Selmar, and Soder, 1984), and the *Weiss Comprehensive Articulation Test* (Weiss, 1980) were compared. According to Garn-Nunn and Martin (1992), the conventional articulation assessments, for the most part, identified the children as disordered, but they did not differentiate severity level. They also did not rate some errors as more severe in terms of reducing intelligibility. The conventional tests made programming for phonological remediation more difficult.

Hodson's *The Assessment of Phonological Processes—Revised* (1986) requires the child to choose and then name 50 three-dimensional stimuli or objects. These words are then analyzed. A spontaneous speech sample is also recorded. Hodson (1986) recommends the use of a specific word list to ensure that a large number of phonological processes are analyzed to be reexamined at a later date. The words are recorded on a data sheet that allows the speech-language clinician to transcribe above the word. Then a grid is completed. This grid divides the phonological processes into classes. The last component is a phonological analysis summary from which an average Phonological Process Percentage-of-Occurrence

Score can be derived, as well as a severity rating and a Phonological Deviancy Score (PDS). The scoring of these responses can be done via the *Computer Analysis of Phonological Processes* (Hodson, 1985).

In one study (Garrett and Moran, 1992), the PDS from *The Assessment of Phonological Processes–Revised* (Hodson, 1986) and the percent consonants correct (PCC) from the *Natural Process Analysis* (Shriberg and Kwiatkowski, 1980) were compared. Both were scored via computer programs. The data suggested that both measures were of similar value in making severity assessments. There was also a high degree of correlation between listener ratings and the PDS and PCC scores. Thus, single-word response tasks can be clinically useful, especially if combined with an analysis of connected speech, as recommended by the authors of the instruments.

Any of the above methods can be used to determine if a child has a phonological disorder. They are also clinically useful in determining intervention targets. According to Hodson (1992a), a phonological assessment instrument should:

1. provide information about the severity of the disorder;
2. provide direction for remediation;
3. provide baseline data for accountability;
4. sample all phonemes in a child's language at least once;
5. give at least 10 opportunities for each major phonological pattern to occur;
6. provide some way to identify a child's target; and
7. be administered in 20 minutes or less.

Phonological evaluation also needs to include all other related areas, such as oral motor skills, hearing acuity, and language proficiency.

Hodson's *The Assessment of Phonological Processes–Revised* (1986) is recommended for use with *Phonobuilding* because it has the elements listed above and because the author gives specific areas to target once remediation is initiated. *Phonobuilding* works very well with the approach of targeting patterns in cycles.

Remediation Guidelines

Terms Defined

The following terms define specific phonological patterns or classes of phonemes. An example of each term is provided.

*   *syllableness*—use of the correct number of syllables in a word. For example, *basket* and *ba ba* would both be correct in terms of syllables if the target word was *basket*.
*   *prevocalic*—refers to a sound that occurs before a vowel. The /m/ in *met* is a prevocalic sound.

10

- *postvocalic*—refers to a sound that follows a vowel. The /t/ in *met* is postvocalic.
- *singleton*—a single sound.
- *consonant sequence*—two or more consonant sounds in a word or between words without an intervening vowel sound. The /tr/ in *train* or the /spr/ in *sprinkle* are consonant sequences; is similar to *consonant cluster* or *blend*s which are consecutive consonants in the same syllable.
- *stridents*—sounds produced by noisy turbulence caused by forceful airflow striking the back of the teeth. The stridents are /f, v, s, z, ʃ, ʒ, ʧ, ʤ/.
- *velars*—consonants produced by arching the back of the tongue so it contacts the soft palate. The velars are /k, g, ŋ/.
- *alveolars*—consonants produced by placing the tongue on or close to the alveolar ridge in the front of the mouth. The alveolars are /t, d, n, l, s, z/.
- *liquids*—consonants for which the articulators make only partial, frictionless approximation. The liquids are /r, l/.
- *glides*—prevocalic consonants produced by rapid tongue movements from a high front or high back tongue arch to the vowel that follows. The glides are /w, j/.
- *nasals*—consonants produced by blocking the oral cavity and emitting the sound through the nose. The nasals are /m, n, ŋ/.
- *stops*—consonant sounds which have a completely occluded airstream /p, t, k, b, d, g/.
- *fricatives*—consonant sounds which have a partially occluded airstream causing continuous noise /f, v, θ, ð, s, z, ʃ, ʒ, h/.
- *affricates*—consonant sounds which have a complete stoppage of the airstream followed by a release of continuous noise /ʧ, ʤ/.
- *vowels*—speech sounds produced with an unobstructed vocal tract.

Developmental Data

There have not been established norms for specific ages at which phonological processes are suppressed (Hodson and Paden, 1991). Some available data suggest that the percentage of occurrence for specific processes decreases as children 1½ years old approach the age of 2½. The phonological processes most likely to be repressed are postvocalic singleton obstruent omission, syllable reduction, velar deviation, and nasal/glide deviation. Other phonological processes are still clearly present in the speech of the 2½ year olds. These are liquid deviations and cluster reduction (Preisser, Hodson, and Paden, 1988).

Certain word structure patterns appear first in most children's speech. These are CV and CVCV patterns. Research also indicates that stops, nasals, and glides are among the first classes of phonemes to emerge in the speech of normally

11

developing children and in children with phonological disorders (Stoel-Gammon and Dunn, 1985).

Hodson (1992b) reports that syllableness in the form of CVCV and VCV patterns is acquired at 18–24 months of age. Word-final consonants are also acquired at that time. At 2–3 years of age, children acquire velars, alveolars, and stridents, including /s/ clusters. The speech of a 3- to 4-year-old is more adult-like; omissions of consonants are rare and simplification processes are suppressed. Prevocalic /l/ is acquired at 2–4 years and prevocalic and postvocalic /r/ is acquired at 3–5 years. By 6–7 years of age, sibilants are perfected (i.e., without lisps).

Determining Intervention Targets

Targeting specific phonological patterns is an important step in planning a child's remediation (Hodson, 1992b). Hodson and Paden (1991) select their intervention targets based on the results obtained from *The Assessment of Phonological Processes–Revised* (Hodson, 1986). Phonological processes needing remediation are those occurring more than 40 percent of the time that the child has the opportunity to use the phonological processes. Stimulability is a critical factor for choosing intervention targets. The child must be ready to produce a specific target.

As recommended by Hodson (1992a), the order of target pattern/phoneme presentation for a child is based on assessment findings, developmental information, as well as phonological research. Voiced final obstruents (/b, d, g, z/) are never targeted for preschoolers because devoicing of final obstruents in word-final position is commonly observed in the utterances of children with normally developing phonology. Hodson (1992b) also specifies that vocalic /l/, /ŋ/, /θ/, /ð/, sibilants, and weak syllables are inappropriate targets for preschoolers.

Hodson (1992b) recommends targeting word-initial liquids during each cycle. The targeting of these sounds early on seems to save years of remediation time. This is especially true for the /r/ sound. Each child's speech processes and patterns must be examined and an individual program suited to the development of intelligible speech for the child must be created.

Phonological Patterns

The following is the hierarchy of potential target patterns/phonemes that Hodson (1992a) most often considers for remediation:

Early Developing Patterns

Syllableness—vowel sequences in compound words (for syllable reduction)

Word-initial consonant singletons—labial glide, nasal, stops (/w, m, b, p/) (for deletion of word-initial consonants)

Postvocalic voiceless stops /p, t, k/ (for deletion of final consonants); nasals /m, n/ (if word-final nasals are lacking)

Posterior/Anterior Contrasts

Velars—word-final /k/ (for fronting or omission of velars); then, word-initial /k, g, h/

Alveolars—word-initial /t, d, n/ (for backing or omission of alveolars)

/s/ Clusters

Word-initial /s/ clusters (/sp/; /sm/ and/or /sn/ if the child has nasals; /st/ if the child has /d/ and /t/; and/or /sk/ if the child produces prevocalic velars)

Word-final /s/ clusters—stop-plus /s/;/ts, ps, ks/

Liquids

Prevocalic liquid—word-initial /l/

Prevocalic liquid—word-initial /r/

Additional Target Patterns—Secondary

Voicing contrasts (prevocalic only)

Vowel contrasts (nondialectal)

Anterior strident singletons /f, s/

Palatal glide /j/

Palatal sibilants /ʃ, ʧ, ʤ/

Postvocalic/syllabic /r/

Word-medial consonants

Word-initial 3-consonant clusters (e.g., /str/)

Additional Target Patterns—Advanced

Complex consonant sequences

Multisyllabicity

Facilitative Phonetic Contexts

The context of the target pattern/phoneme within a word is also important to consider. Some phonemes seem to facilitate the production of other phonemes. These facilitative phonetic contexts as well as a child's idiosyncratic ability to produce a target within a specific word need to be considered.

Kent (1982) lists three factors to consider when examining the phonetic context of a specific sound to determine if it is facilitating—the position of the sound in the word, the stress pattern of the word or syllable, and the neighboring or adjacent sounds. Based on his review of various studies, Kent (1982) suggests several principles to consider:

- Present the error sound in a stressed syllable.
- Present /r/ sounds initially in /dr/, /tr/, and /gr/ blends.

- Present /s/ in medial or final-word position instead of word-initial position (except for word-initial /s/ clusters /sp/, /st/, and /sn/).
- Present fricatives in word-final position.
- Present /s/ clusters in /sp/, /st/, and /sn/ blends in word-initial position.

Based on Kent's (1982) findings and because of complexity aspects, Hodson and Paden (1991) use only monosyllabic targets during cycle 1.

Phonological Cycles Approach

Hodson and Paden's (1991) approach identifies the phonological processes in a child's speech. The child's processes determine the pattern targeted in remediation. Individual phonemes are used to focus on the target pattern, so words are chosen that contain both the target sounds and target patterns. Individual phonemes are used only as a means to an end. Basic to their approach is maintaining the interest of the child while continuing to move from phoneme to phoneme and from pattern to pattern (Hodson and Paden, 1991).

In Hodson and Paden's model, phonological patterns are targeted in cycles. A certain criterion of correct responses is not necessary for moving on to the next pattern, rather the goal is to achieve as nearly as possible, 100% accuracy on the carefully selected production-practice words. (Determining intervention targets is discussed beginning on page 12.) The use of cycles began after experiments with children having severely impaired speech intelligibility revealed that these children improved their speech when they were introduced to a new pattern and then allowed to internalize this new pattern over the course of a few months (Hodson and Paden, 1991). A cycle is the sequential targeting of several patterns over time.

Cycle 1

Cycles are on a time frame; each cycle takes from 6 to 20 weeks of 1-hour remediation sessions weekly. The length of a cycle depends on the number of patterns needing to be targeted and the number of stimulable sounds within the target pattern (Hodson and Paden, 1991). For example, if consonant sequence reduction was a phonological process identified in the child's speech, initial /s/ blends could be one of the targets during cycle 1. Thus, the phonological process used by the child is consonant sequence reduction, the target pattern is consonant sequences, and the sounds used to elicit the pattern are /s/ blends.

Depending on the child's progress, this pattern of consonant sequences could be addressed for 2 to 6 weeks of 1-hour remediation sessions. The shorter amount of time would be used if the child quickly learned the new pattern or if the child was unable to use the new pattern and was frustrated. The greater amount of time would reflect that the child had other patterns targeted and was stimulable for several phonemes within the patterns.

Within cycle 1, different /s/ blends would be targeted. The emphasis might begin with /st/, move to /sk/, and then /sp/ before a new phonological pattern would be addressed. Specific phonemes are addressed for 60 minutes. This can be done in one session of 1 hour, two 30-minute sessions, or three 20-minute sessions (Hodson and Paden, 1991). The next phonological pattern to be targeted within cycle 1 would be chosen and addressed for 1 to 2 weeks of 1-hour remediation sessions. Once all of the child's phonological processes have been targeted, cycle 2 begins.

Cycle 2

In cycle 2, the phonological processes addressed in cycle 1 that are still in error are "recycled" (Hodson and Paden, 1991). New patterns may be used to remediate these phonological processes. For example, the target pattern of consonant sequences could focus on stop-plus-liquid sounds such as /pl/ and /kl/. Within each cycle, the two main components of each session are intensive auditory stimulation and the production of as many correct responses as can be achieved in a natural environment.

Component One: Auditory Stimulation

Auditory stimulation involves giving the child as many auditory cues as possible. Hodson and Paden (1991) suggest reading lists of 10–15 target words containing the target pattern/phoneme for 2 minutes at the beginning and end of each session. This list may or may not include the target production-practice words (i.e., those that will be produced by the child [see page 16]). The use of amplification so the child's auditory channel is truly stimulated is also recommended. The child can then be asked to repeat the target phonemes.

Component Two: Natural Environment

Component two, producing sounds in a natural environment, refers to activities in which the child responds to a stimulus when producing target words but is not engaged in drill-type activities (e.g., the child could be engaged in a guessing game, finding and naming pictures, or responding to questions when producing target words or phonemes).

Hodson and Paden (1991) recommend that remediation involve activities designed to keep the child's interest and to facilitate correct production of sound patterns. Reading is recommended for facilitating correct patterns in older children. Reading material that is at a lower level than the child's actual reading level should be chosen so that the emphasis is on sound production and not on the reading process. The professional and child can take turns reading the book or choose parts and read as if it were a script for a play. The material can also be read silently and then the speech-language clinician can question the child about what was read. Another method of using books is to discuss the text or pictures after the material has been reviewed. *Phonobuilding* stories would be appropriate to use in this way.

How to Use *Phonobuilding*

General Procedures

Once the specific pattern to be developed has been chosen, a target sound to facilitate the use of the pattern needs to be selected. The story that corresponds to the target pattern and sound is identified from the List of Stories on pages 27–28. The following steps are guidelines to effective remediation.

1. Selecting a Story

After a thorough phonological evaluation, the speech-language clinician should select the story that contains the target pattern (i.e., the pattern that the child needs to develop) and the target sound (i.e., the stimulable phonemes within the pattern).

2. Selecting the Target Words

Each story contains 10 target words that are listed preceding the story. These target words are used as the production-practice words in the Production-Practice Activities (see page 17). Not all of these words provide the most facilitative phonetic context for the correct production of the target pattern/phoneme. Consequently, the target words are divided into two lists at the beginning of each story. The list called "Cycle 1" contains those target words with the most facilitative phonetic context for correct production of the target pattern/phoneme and which are best for cycle 1. The other list, called "Later Cycles," contains words whose phonetic context is less facilitating and would be more appropriate for cycles 2, or 3, etc.

During cycle 1, use only those words with a facilitative phonetic context for correct production of the target pattern/phoneme. The speech-language clinician should read the pictographs of words for later cycles when using *Phonobuilding* stories during cycle 1. During subsequent cycles, probe with the "Later Cycles" words to see if the child is ready to use them (i.e., the target sound is stimulable).

The speech-language clinician should also read the morphological markers following "Cycle 1" words since the addition of the markers changes the phonetic context of some words. For example, the word "ski" provides a facilitative phonetic context for production of word-initial /s/ blends but the word "skiing," which occurs in the story, is multisyllabic and is less facilitative for correct production of the target pattern/phoneme. In this case, the child should read the pictograph as "ski" and the speech-language clinician should quickly follow with "ing."

Next to each word in the lists is a frequency-of-occurrence number in parentheses. This number indicates how many times the target word is represented in the story.

16

3. Organizing Materials

The chosen story should be duplicated for the child to use and take home. Each story is preceded by reproducible illustrations of the pictographs in the story. These illustrations should be duplicated on heavier stock paper and cut apart to be used as cards for the activities described in step 7 of this discussion. For some of the activities, two sets of cards are needed. The pictographs in the story and the pictograph cards can be colored by the speech-language pathologist before use or by the child during auditory stimulation.

For several of the stories, the target word is a color word and is represented by open circles. These need to be shaded in with the appropriate colors before using.

4. Reading the Story

During the session, the professional reads the story to the child, emphasizing the target words and pointing to the pictographs as they are named. This aids phonological remediation by enhancing ear training (Hodson and Paden, 1991). The child's initial exposure to a new sound is within a language context.

5. Reading the Pictographs

The speech-language clinician then introduces the child to pictographs from the story by reading them. Only "Cycle 1" target words should be used during cycle 1. During subsequent cycles, "Cycle 1" words can be emphasized as well as target words from the "Later Cycles" list. The child's full attention is now on the specific target words and their visual association.

6. Drawing Pictographs

The child is then asked to draw his or her own pictographs that emphasize the target words from the story. This drawing continues from session to session until all the target words are drawn. Only three to four pictographs should be drawn per session (Hodson and Paden, 1991). Index cards work best, and the pictographs need to be labeled with the target word. While the child draws the pictographs, the meaning of the word or uses of the word can be described by the speech-language clinician. This enhances sound development and expands vocabulary skills. If drawing is not appropriate for the child, the pictograph cards from the story may be used for the activities that follow in step 7.

7. Production-Practice Activities

The child can use the pictograph cards in motivational activities. Many of the following activity ideas are commonly used by speech-language clinicians:

17

- **Go fish**—Attach a thin magnet to each pictograph or a paper clip and create a fishing pole with a magnet at one end. Place the cards on the table or the floor. Have the child "fish" for the cards and name them as they are found.

- **Match games**—Using the cards from the stories and the child's cards, play various matching games. Have the child name the cards as they are chosen.

- **Memory**—Select from three to five of the child's cards. Name the cards for the child and have the child repeat the names. Ask the child to remember where each card is. Then turn the cards over. Name a pictograph and have the child find it and name it.

Additional ideas suggested by Hodson and Paden (1983) follow:

- **Hide-and-seek**—Hide the child's cards in the room and have the child find the cards and then name the pictograph, with or without a model, using appropriately produced sounds. A variation to this activity would be to have the child hide the cards and provide clues to the professional. Discussing the words while simultaneously emphasizing the target sounds is effective.

- **Flashlight game**—Turn off the bright lights in the room and leave on a small light or slightly open the door for light. Place the cards on the floor in an open area. Give a flashlight to the child and ask him or her to locate a specific pictograph. When it is found, have the child name it. Continue this process until all the cards are found.

- **Toss or roll**—Place the cards on the table or on the floor and have the child name a card at which he or she aims a penny or a small ball. Have the child toss the penny or roll the ball. If the target card is hit, have the child name the pictograph and get the card. Continue this process until all the cards are gone.

Other ideas include:

- **Basket pick**—Place all cards in a basket. Hold the basket slightly above the child's head and have the child choose a card. Have the child name each card as it is chosen and continue until all cards have been picked.

- **Dice toss**—Number cards from one to six. (If using less than six cards, assign two numbers to one or more cards; if using more than six cards, two or more cards may share the same number allowing the child to name both cards when the number is tossed, or use two dice.) Have the child toss a die and name the card corresponding to the number showing on the die.

8. Continuing Remediation

During subsequent sessions, the child participates in the story by reading the pictographs while the story is being read. The child may not be ready to produce specific target words until cycle 2. Eventually, the child should be able to name all of the pictographs during story reading. The child who can name all of the pictographs with correctly produced sounds should be encouraged to retell the story to peers, family members, or the speech-language clinician using his or her own pictographs.

9. Ending the Session

At the end of each session, all of the pictographs from the story should be named by the speech-language clinician, with the target sounds emphasized. This, again, enhances auditory awareness. The speech-language clinician can use the child's pictographs if they have all been drawn or the duplicated illustrations from *Phonobuilding*. This ear training should last approximately 2 minutes (Hodson and Paden, 1991).

10. Practicing at Home

The speech-language clinician determines the child's level and thoroughly discusses it with parents or caregivers or provides clearly written directions for them to follow. The parents or caregivers should be aware of the steps through which the child needs to progress before he or she will be ready to say the words or to use new words in conversational speech. The child's cards should be kept in a communication folder with a copy of the story. The folder should be sent home after each session.

The parental or caregiver involvement with the child should mirror what is occurring in remediation. Initially, the parents or caregivers use auditory awareness techniques such as reading the pictographs or reading the story and simultaneously emphasizing the target words. When the child is ready to say the words, the child can practice repeating them. The next step would be to name the pictographs spontaneously. Then the child is ready to help the parents or caregivers read the story by reading the pictographs as the parents or caregivers read the words. Parents or caregivers should be cautioned to stop practice at any time if the child is producing more than approximately 20 percent of target sounds in error. The final step is to have the child retell the story using his or her own picture cards.

Monitoring Progress

To monitor progress, the speech-language clinician should list the phonological processes that the child used during the initial evaluation. If *The Assessment of Phonological Processes—Revised* (Hodson, 1986) was used, the Phonological Process Percentage-of-Occurrence Score and Severity Rating sheet that is included with the assessment could be used. To calculate a Phonological Process Percentage-of-Occurrence Score, determine how many times a specific phonological process had the opportunity to be present in the assessment words. Then determine how many times the child used the phonological process. Divide the total number of actual occurrences of the phonological process by the number of opportunities for its occurrence to determine a percentage score. For example, if there were 10 words with more than one syllable, the child had 10 opportunities to use the phonological process of syllable reduction. If the child produced 6 of these words with only one syllable, then the percentage of occurrence of the process of syllable reduction would be 60 percent.

Hodson and Paden (1991) recommend addressing any phonological process that exceeds 40 percent, except for glides, where the cutoff is 70 percent. After all the phonological patterns are targeted in cycle 1, the speech-language clinician should readminister the initial assessment to determine what progress was made. Carryover is not to be expected until cycle 2 or 3. Hodson and Paden (1991) also recommend "speech vacations" during which the child is to have a complete break from practicing speech sounds. In the schools, these breaks occur naturally. For clinics or hospitals, short speech vacations need to be built into the remediation schedule.

If the speech-language clinician is not using Hodson's *The Assessment of Phonological Processes–Revised* (1986), a list of phonological processes used by a child, with their percentages of occurrence, needs to be made and used for comparisons between cycles to monitor progress.

Using *Phonobuilding* to Develop Communication Skills

The stories written for *Phonobuilding* can be used to develop a variety of communication skills. These include:

- vocabulary development
- word retrieval
- reasoning
- question comprehension
- emergent literacy skills
- story retelling
- written language skills

Vocabulary Development

The use of *Phonobuilding* for expanding vocabulary knowledge can follow procedures applied to many types of literature in which the vocabulary words unfamiliar to the child are examined. It is best if the child hears the entire story read first, so all the words are presented in context. The pictographs should be pointed to by the speech-language clinician as the story is read. Unfamiliar words can be written down by the child or the professional. Forms for this process are provided in Appendix A. The unfamiliar word is listed in the left column, and the child draws a small picture to the right of the word. In the third column, the child writes an explanation of the picture; the speech-language clinician helps with this task as needed. In the far right column, the child writes a sentence that uses the word correctly or dictates a sentence to the speech-language clinician to write. Not more than three vocabulary words should be emphasized per session for younger children. The vocabulary sheet should be duplicated so the child can bring one copy home to be reviewed with parents or caregivers. The speech-language clinician keeps one copy to review in subsequent intervention sessions. The number of rows can be varied according to the level of the student. For primary-level students (i.e., pre-kindergarten through grade 2), there should be no more than three rows, as in the blank vocabulary sheet on page 255. For older students, six rows work well. Synonyms, antonyms, or multiple meanings of the target word could also be incorporated into this activity by adapting the form (i.e., adding columns or rows to allow for new information).

Sample Vocabulary Sheet

word	sketch	explanation	word used in a sentence
block		A space in a city To prevent entry	I walked around the block. The chair blocked the door.

The use of *Phonobuilding* stories to enhance vocabulary works well in a group setting. The story is read to the group. If the group is small enough so that everyone can see the pictographs, only one copy of the story is needed. If the group is larger, children should have their own copies of the selected story. Duplicate a vocabulary sheet for each child. If specific words have been chosen in advance, these can be written in the appropriate column. Discussion of the words, drawing of pictures, and the writing of explanations and sentences all need to be done in a step-by-step fashion. When all of the words that the educator, speech-language clinician, or students have identified as difficult have been listed, sketched, and discussed, the story can be read again so the words are repeated in a meaningful context.

Word Retrieval

Improving word-retrieval skills can also be a part of the remediation process. The child can be given opportunities to participate in "cloze" procedures, which are similar to sentence completion or fill-in-the-blank tasks. The speech-language clinician reads the printed story text and the child fills in the blanks by reading the pictographs. This can be done on a variety of levels. To make the task easier, the speech-language clinician can say the names of the pictographs to the child and have the child repeat them. Giving the child cues about the phonetic makeup of the words (i.e., "These all start with /sp/") would also make the task easier (Wiig and Semel, 1980).

Visual imagery is already built into this task through the use of pictographs. Visual imagery is a known strategy for helping students who have word-naming and retrieval problems (Wiig and Semel, 1980). This strategy could be discussed in terms of teaching the child to make pictures in his or her mind to recall specific words. For younger children, actually drawing pictures may be necessary before the concept of creating visual images will be understood.

Reasoning

Reasoning skills (i.e., problem solving, hypothetical thinking, and inferring cause and effect) can be enhanced through predicting outcomes for a story, creating alternative actions for the characters in a story, discussing inferences, and answering "why" questions to ascertain cause and effect.

The best way to approach reasoning tasks is to decide which aspect of reasoning is to be addressed. If inference is the target, then enough of the story should be read so predictions can be made about the outcome of the story. For creating alternative actions, hypothesizing, or answering "why" questions, the entire story needs to be read to the child (or by the child) and then discussed.

Question Comprehension

Comprehension of oral and written material can be enhanced through questioning students about the material (Merritt, 1989; Schory, 1990). Strategies to teach students who have difficulty with question comprehension include:

1. telling students what information needs to be discovered from a specific story or a specific paragraph;
2. giving the students the question before the story is read;
3. asking students to use visual imagery cues while listening; and
4. having students take notes or draw a picture to aid memory retention.

After one or more of these strategies has been discussed, the story should be read by or to the student. The appraisal of these strategies as being effective or not effective is important for helping each student know what works for him or her.

Emergent Literacy Skills

Emergent literacy skills, or readiness for reading, can be enhanced using *Phonobuilding*. Children can read the pictographs and take part in the reading process, thereby learning front-to-back, left-to-right, and top-to-bottom progression; the concept of a word; and the concepts of a beginning, middle, and end to a story. Children learn that they can read using the pictographs that represent written words. They then use matching and memory of phonetic cues to begin to read the words that replace the pictographs as the professional reads the rest of the story.

Story Retelling

The *Phonobuilding* stories lend themselves very well to story retelling or story generation using the provided pictures. This task can be used for diagnostic purposes or to enhance a child's narrative skills. Merritt (1989) suggests that using story retelling for diagnostic purposes often provides a speech-language clinician with a longer speech sample, greater use of clauses, and more complete episodes than asking a child to make up a story. A story model appears to guide both language-impaired and nonimpaired children in organizing story content into complete episodes (Merritt, 1989).

The speech-language clinician can also use one storytelling task as a baseline against which to measure progress. Narrated stories can be assessed through a narrative analysis or through a specific story grammar process as outlined in *Storybuilding* (Hutson-Nechkash, 1990).

Children develop narrative skills by being read stories as well as by telling stories. Hutson-Nechkash (1990) describes narrations as:

1. containing extended units of text;
2. having story markers, including an introduction, closing, and proper sequences of events; and
3. presenting information without listener input or questions for clarification.

Hutson-Nechkash (1990) clearly outlines the acquisition of narrative skills. This sequence is reprinted with permission in Appendix B.

Children can improve their narrative skills by retelling the stories in *Phonobuilding*. Viewing the story with pictographs as they retell it may help simplify the task, as the pictographs can help with proper sequencing and presenting of events within each story.

Written Language Skills

Written language skills can be addressed by having children rewrite endings to the *Phonobuilding* stories. Depending on the age of the child, these story endings can be written by the child or dictated to the professional, who in turn does the writing. The pictographs can also be used to help children create their

23

own stories. Mixing pictographs from different stories can lead to many creative, new stories. Initially, children can dictate if the actual writing process seems to be a hindrance, but as they become more fluent at creating stories, they can begin to assume the actual writing process. Written work, especially the child's own work, lends itself to editing. This could include an examination of syntax, word usage, and cohesion of ideas. Teaching expansion of written sentences through the use of the question words *why, when, where,* and *how* is also appropriate.

Tips for Implementing *Phonobuilding*

Use with Groups

Speech-language clinicians are able to use this resource with groups of children. For children developing phonological skills, it is helpful if the children in the group have the same patterns as targets. Groups of two to three children are ideal. The groups can be more heterogeneous if other language skills are being developed.

Heterogenous Groups

When addressing communication skills (other than phonological remediation), larger groups can be accommodated. If the story is being read and the pictographs used, the group needs to be small enough so that all of the students can clearly see the pictures, or multiple copies of the stories need to be distributed.

Creating More Stories

Creating more stories using specific target words can be done by the professional or the children. This can often be done by gathering a group of specific words and then selecting a known story on which to model the new story. For example, a story could be written as a variation on "Hansel and Gretel," using the idea of two children becoming lost in the woods.

Auditory Bombardment

For phonological development, the concept of auditory stimulation is crucial. The targeted story needs to be read at the beginning of each session. The target words also need to be modeled by the professional. The reading of the words must also be done at the end of the session. For an hour-long session, 2 minutes of auditory stimulation at the onset and at the close of the session are recommended (Hodson and Paden, 1991).

Phonobuilding Stories

The *Phonobuilding* stories that follow are based on Hodson's (1992a) recommended remediation targets. The stories are listed according to the phonological pattern/phoneme targeted within it. Professionals should be creative in using "Later Cycles" target words for secondary and advanced patterns.

List of Stories

Patterns	Title

Early Developing Patterns

Syllableness..The Keyhole Adventure

Prevocalic Singletons—Labial Glide, Nasal, Stop

Word-initial /w/ ....The Witch's Ride

Word-initial /m/.................................Min and the Men on the Moon

Word-initial /p/ ....The Pup Paints

Postvocalic Singletons—Voiceless Stops

Word-final /t/ ....Nuts About Nuts

Word-final /k/ ....Oak Tree Listens

Word-final /p/ ....Soup Thieves

Posterior/Anterior Contrasts

Velars

Word-final /k/ ....Help for Mike

Word-initial /k/ ....Cookies for the King

Word-initial /k/ ....Come Follow Me

Alveolars

Word-initial /t/ ....Two Ants Travel

Word-initial /n/ ....Necktie Finds a New Home

/s/ Clusters

Word-initial /s/ clusters

/sp/ ....Spoon and the Funny Spice

/st/ ....Wishing on a Star

/sk/ ....Skip Dreams

Word-final—Stop-plus /s/ ....Pups' Vacation Planning

Liquids

Word-initial /l/ ....Playmates for Lynn

Word-initial /l/ blends ....Santa Saves the Sleeping Baby ✓

Word-initial /r/ ....A Rest for Rattlesnake

Secondary Target Patterns

Anterior strident singletons

Word-initial /f/ ....Fox and the Fat Fish

Word-initial /s/ ....Sam's Magnificent Scene

Word-medial consonants ....Selective "Later Cycles" target words

Advanced Target Patterns

Complex consonant sequences

Word-final /st/ blends ....Fox Goes to First Grade ✓

Multisyllabicity...Selective "Later Cycles" target words ✓

The Keyhole Adventure

Target Sound: syllableness

Target Pattern: syllableness

Target Words

Cycle 1

cowboy (9)   sunlight (2)   iceberg (4)

footballs (2)   meatballs (5)   highway (5)

keyhole (8)   seashells (3)

Later Cycles

donkey (11)   turkey (9)

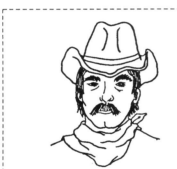

cowboy

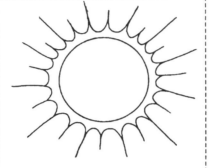

sunlight

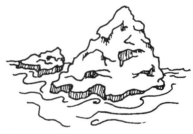

iceberg

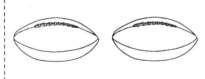

footballs

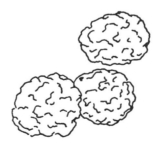

meatballs

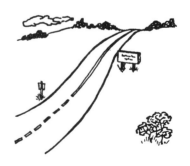

highway

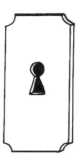

keyhole

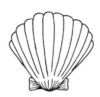

seashells

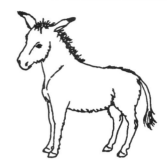

donkey

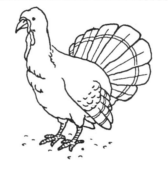

turkey

The Keyhole Adventure

Once upon a time, there was a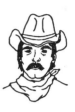

who had a pet . The 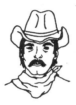 and the

 would ride on their 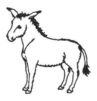 whenever

they needed to go on a journey. One day,

the 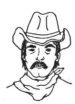 and the 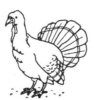 hopped on the

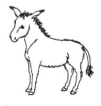 and said, "Take us on an adventure."

So the 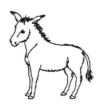 started off down the 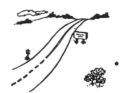 .

They traveled through several towns, up some

mountains, and down into some valleys,

but they did not find any adventure.

The 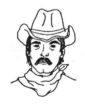 was becoming tired, the

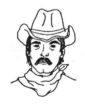 was becoming stiff, and the

was becoming bored. "Where will this

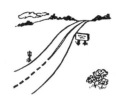 lead us?" asked the 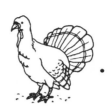. "I am

bored from the lack of adventure."

"Just wait and see," promised the

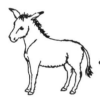. On and on they plodded down the

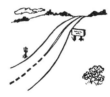. Finally, they met an interesting

sight just ahead of them. The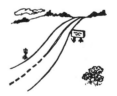

ended and there was a giant-sized 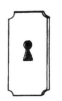.

"Look at that 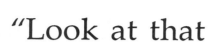 ," said the 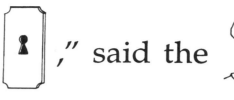 . "Is

there a key big enough to fit in that ?"

he asked.

"No," said the 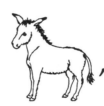 , "there's no key.

That is for us to pass through. Then

we will surely have an adventure."

The , the 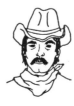 , and the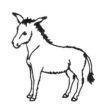

were more than a little bit afraid as they

passed out of the 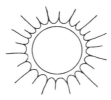 and into the dark

 .

Once they passed through the ,

the 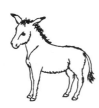 stepped onto an 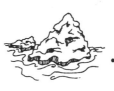 . They

began floating down a very quiet river.

The 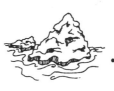 was cold, but the surrounding

air was warm. They floated through the

darkness, and then they heard some

music.

Some 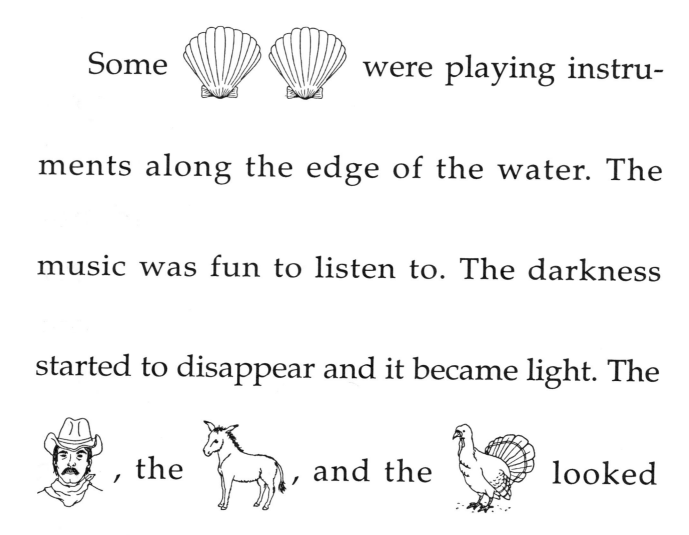 were playing instru-

ments along the edge of the water. The

music was fun to listen to. The darkness

started to disappear and it became light. The

, the , and the looked

around. This was quite an adventure!

The 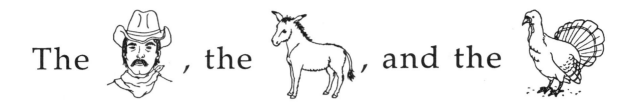 , the , and the

were becoming hungry. They asked the

musical 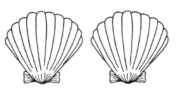 if there was food for

them to eat. The 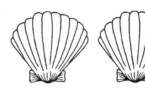 did not

answer, but soon some 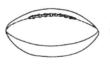 with

arms handed them some . The

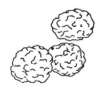 smelled delicious. They each took

a bite. The were delicious. The

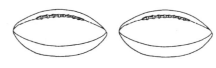 served them many 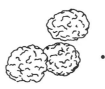 .

The were a wonderful feast.

Soon the 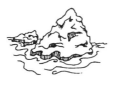 began floating

backward. Back to the the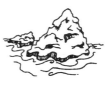

took them. It took them back through the

 , back onto the 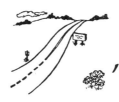 , and back into

the . The 🫏 , the 🤠 , and the

🦃   agreed that they had quite an

adventure.

The Witch's Ride

Target Sound: word-initial /w/   **Target Pattern:** prevocalic singletons (labial glide)

Target Words

Cycle 1

wheat (7)   one (4)   week (3)

west (2)   whale (12) witch (13)

white (3)   walk (3)   waves (4)

Later Cycles

window (2)

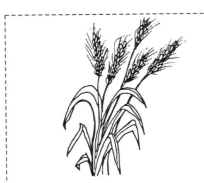

wheat

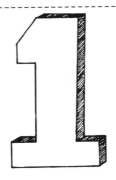

one

week

west

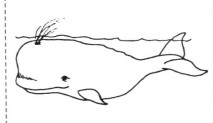

whale

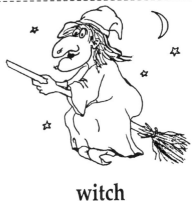

witch

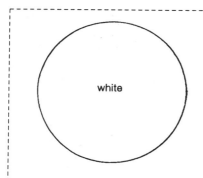

white

white

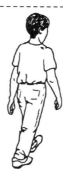

walk

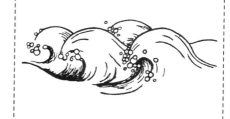

waves

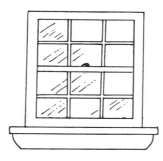

window

The Witch's Ride

Once upon a time, there was a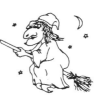

who lived in the 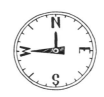 . She was not a

wicked 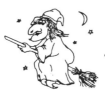 . This 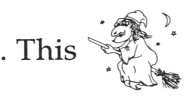 lived on a farm

near an ocean, where she raised .

When she was not busy, she loved to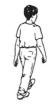

near the ocean to watch a special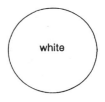

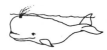 who was her friend.

 day, the 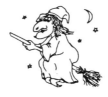 looked out her

 and saw the 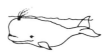 come very

close to the shore. She looked at her

calendar. It was Wednesday, and she had

no plans or appointments for that day of

the .

The 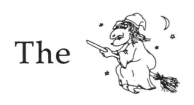 decided to 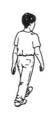 down to

the shore to talk to the . It was a very

windy day, and the ocean was full of

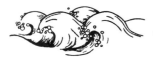. The 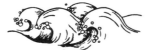 splashing on the

shore created a (white) foam. The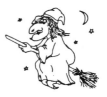

took off her shoes so she could 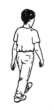 into

the water to speak to the 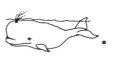.

"Hello," said the 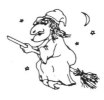 . "I have har-

vested my and I took it to the miller

last . Yesterday, I baked some

bread and cooled it by my . Would

you like some?" asked the 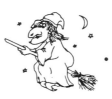 .

"Yes", said the 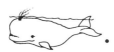 .

Magically, loaf of fresh

bread appeared in the 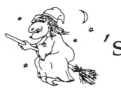 's hands.

"Why don't you bring your 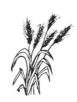 bread

with you and come to a tea party that some

of my 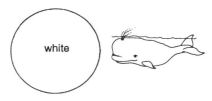 friends are having out at sea?

Hop on my back," said the 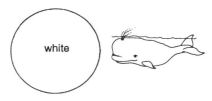.

The 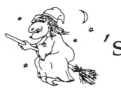 climbed onto the back of

the 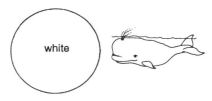 and they headed ,

47

out to sea. On the way, they saw porpoises

and dolphins dancing and playing in the

. They saw some friendly sharks

and not-so-friendly shark.

In the middle of the ocean, there was a

whole school of s. They were having

a tea party. They used seashells for plates

and cups. The s made tea from a

magic brew of foam from the 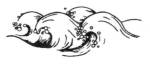 and

a few grains of sand. It was wonderful. The

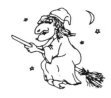 shared her bread with them.

Everyone had a great time at the tea

party. The tea was wonderful and the

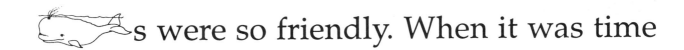s were so friendly. When it was time

for the 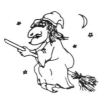 to return home,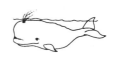

said, "We meet every Wednesday. I hope to

see you next 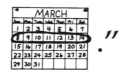 ."

"I would love to come," said the 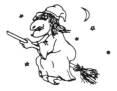 .

"I will bring more 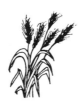 bread."

Min and the Men on the Moon

Target Sound: word-initial /m/   **Target Pattern:** prevocalic singletons (nasal)

Target Words

Cycle 1		
moon (9)	mouth (2)	milk (3)
more (3)	meat (3)	men (8)
Min (15)	man (5)	

Later Cycles
minutes (3)
machines (5)

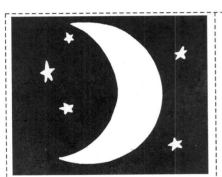

moon

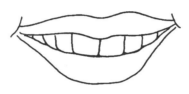

mouth

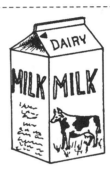

milk

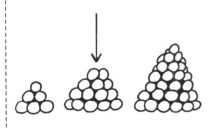

more

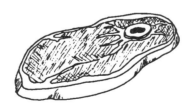

meat

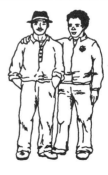

men

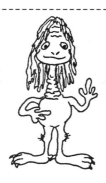

Min

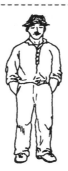

man

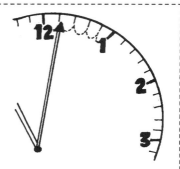

minutes

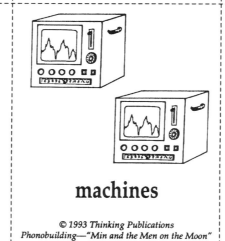

machines

Min and the Men on the Moon

Once upon a time, there was a creature

who lived on the 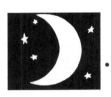. His name was

. One morning, saw a rocket

ship speeding toward him. He moved

behind his house made of 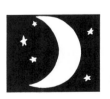 rocks.

 saw the rocket orbit, and then a

small craft landed on his 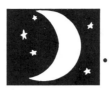. Two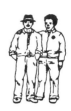

climbed out of the small craft.

The first thing the two space 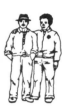 did

was try to move. They seemed to float

with each step they took. One space

planted a red, white, and blue flag on the

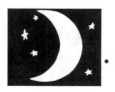. noticed the stars and stripes

on the flag.

The space 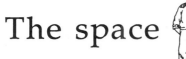 then began to collect

rocks and dust. They put these items into

their spacecraft. did not understand

why they collected those things. He

watched them for several 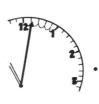 .

The space 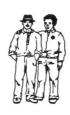 then went aboard their

spacecraft to have a snack of and

. All of their food and drink was in

packages. crept closer to see what

they were doing. He had never before seen

anyone put food in his . He had

never seen or . One space

said, "I would like some 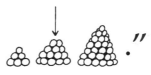."

"I think there is 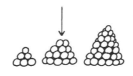 and

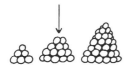 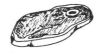 over there," said the other

space 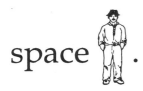 .

The 🌙 creature was very curious.

He moved closer and closer. Now he could

see that each space 🧑 wore clothes. The

material looked soft and flexible. On their

feet were boots, and they both wore pants

and shirts. One even wore something

on his head.

After several of staring into

the spacecraft, noticed all of the

  in there. He wished he knew

how these   worked.

The two space 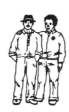 in the spacecraft

58

were startled by a noise. was entering

their craft. They said, "Hello! Who are you?"

There was no response. walked

over to the . He wanted to press

the buttons and pull on the levers.

The space 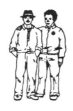 were curious about this

strange, little fellow with the long, yellow

hair and small body. "Can you help me?"

 asked. "I want to turn on these

 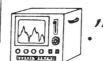."

 did not talk with his . He

moved his hands and words came out.

The space 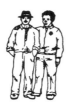 talked to about

their . They talked for several

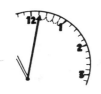. Then said, "Where do you

come from?"

The space 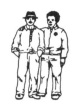 pointed to a planet.

"That is Earth. We call the place where you

live the 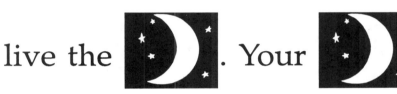. Your circles around

our Earth. Some people claim that there is a

 on the . They must be speaking

about you, . It is time for us to go

back to the Earth. Would you like to come

61

with us?"

"No, thank you. But I would like to visit

with you the next time you come back to

the 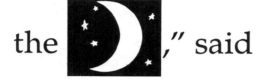 ," said .

The Pup Paints

Target Sound: word-initial /p/   **Target Pattern:** prevocalic singletons (stop)

Target Words

Cycle 1   *Later Cycles*

pup (10)   pin (2)   pail (4)   purple (9)   paper (4)   picture (4)

paste (2)   pour (2)   paint (17)

pink (8)

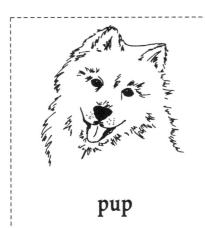

pup

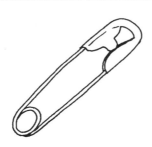

pin

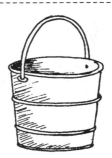

pail

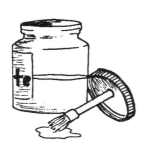

paste

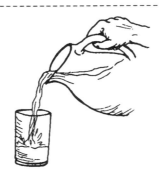

pour

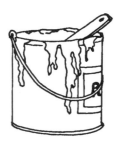

paint

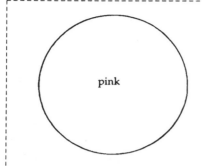

pink

pink

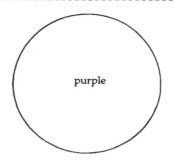

purple

purple

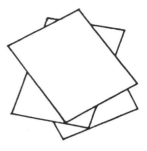

paper

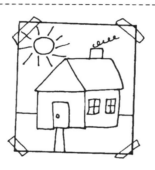

picture

The Pup Paints

Once upon a time, there was a little

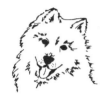 who loved to . Her mother

bought her an easel, 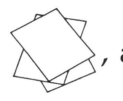 , a brush,

and some 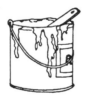 . The 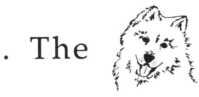 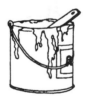ed

s every day. Her mother would

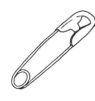 all of her s on the wall. Soon

65

the became bored with her

 brush, her s, and her s.

She stopped having her mother her

 s on the wall.

One day, the 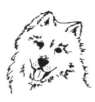 asked her mother if

she could use her father's large brush

and his can of 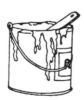 to 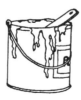 the outside

of the house.

"What color will you the house?"

asked her mother.

"I think I will it 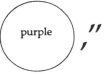," said the

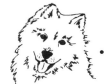. "Yes, with 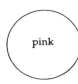 trim would

be wonderful."

Her mother thought for a minute. Then

she said, "I will give you two 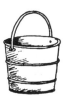s. You

may water in them and I will give

you a brush. Then you can pretend

to the house  and ."

"Well, I think 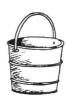s with water in

them will be fine," said the 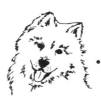.

The found a  and a

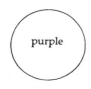 . She ed water in each

one. Then she took two of her father's large

 brushes and pretended to the

house. She worked for a long time on this

project. When she was finished, she

thought the house really looked quite nice

in (purple) and (pink).

Then the 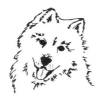 had a new idea. She

went into the house. She found some

scissors, some , and some 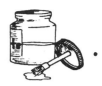.

The was white, but her real

set and her brushes soon turned the

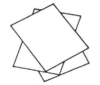 and . The 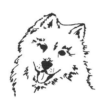 cut

out a shape that looked like a house.

Then she cut out shapes that looked

like windows. She ed the

windows on the house. Now the

 had a real and house.

It was beautiful.

71

Nuts About Nuts

Target Sound: word-final /t/   **Target Pattern:** postvocalic singletons (voiceless stops)

Target Words

Cycle 1			Later Cycles
Nate (13)	nut (9)	boat (17)	
seat (2)	night (2)	eat (6)	
front (3)	sit (2)	fat (3)	
	right (2)		

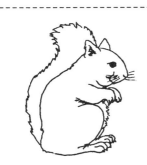

Nate

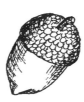

nut

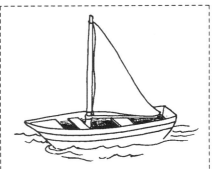

boat

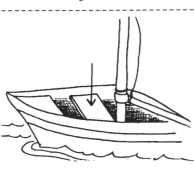

seat

night

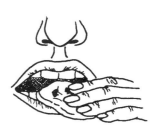

eat

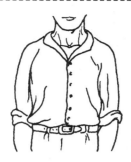

front

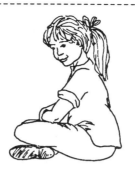

sit

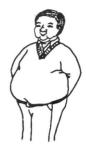

fat

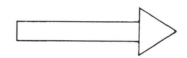

right

Nuts About Nuts

There was a squirrel named 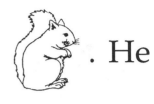 . He

was fluffy and cute. 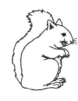 loved to

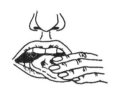 s, and he loved to ride on

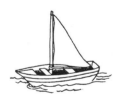 s. But he had trouble finding 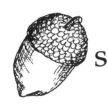 s

to 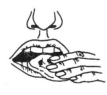 and 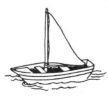 s to ride in.

One day, 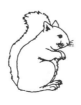 was walking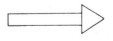

by a lake. He saw a 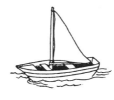 full of 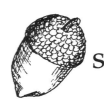s.

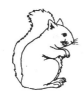 wanted to go for a ride in that

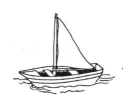, but he could not. The owner was

in the 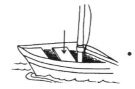. thought he

must be guarding his 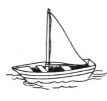 full of 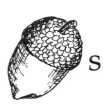s.

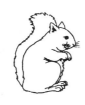 decided to 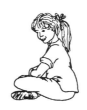 and wait until

it was late, and then maybe the owner

would go away. 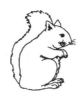 waited and waited,

thinking about riding on that 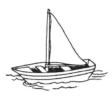 with

a 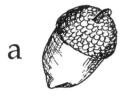 in each hand.

The day turned to , and the man

in the 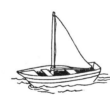 became hungry. He went to

a nearby restaurant to get something to

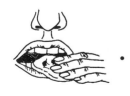 . 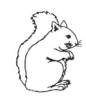 jumped onto the 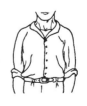 of

77

the 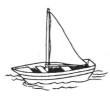 . He began to crack the 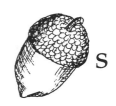 s

and to put them into his mouth as quickly

as possible.

 kept 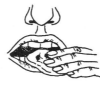 ing and 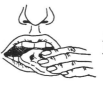 ing.

He began to get a stomachache, so he

decided to 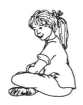 down. But he kept

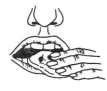 ing. Then 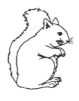 heard a noise. He

looked up. The 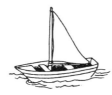 owner was coming

back to his 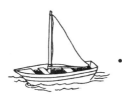 .

The squirrel tried to jump off the

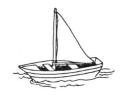 , but he could not move. He had

grown too 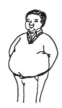 to move. The man looked

at his 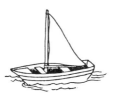 . The s were almost

gone. Then he looked at 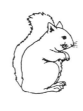 . He began to laugh. The poor squirrel was so 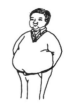 .

"Get off my 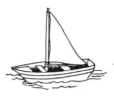 , you 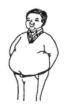 squirrel,"

said the man. 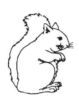 tried to crawl off the

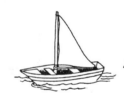 , but he could not.

The man said, "Thank you for getting

all of those s off my 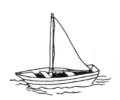 . I was

wondering how I could get rid of them."

80

The man pointed to a walnut tree. "The

s fell from that tree last ," he

said.

The man had an idea. He said, "I would

like you to stay on my 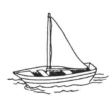 . You can be

in charge of keeping the 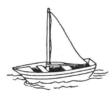 clean. We

will make a good team."

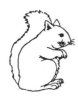 smiled a tiny little smile. Then he

81

fell asleep ⟹ on the 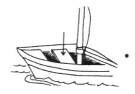 .

Oak Tree Listens

Target Sound: word-final /k/   **Target Pattern:** postvocalic singletons (voiceless stops)

Target Words

Cycle 1			Later Cycles		
back (6)	peek (2)	dark (2)	cheek (5)	seek (2)	sock (3)
oak (6)	book (2)		look (2)	neck (7)	

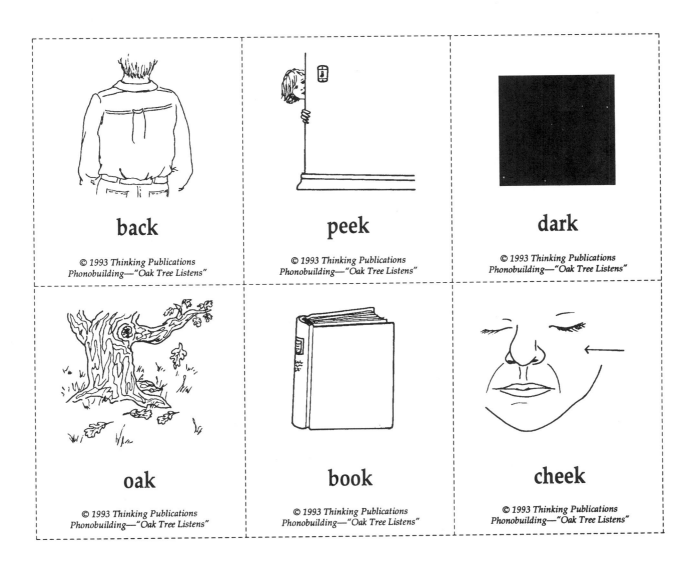

back

peek

dark

oak

book

cheek

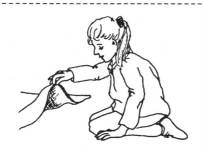

seek

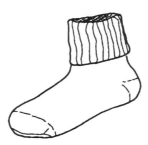

sock

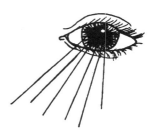

look

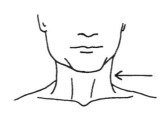

neck

Oak Tree Listens

Once upon a time, there was a little boy.

It was a hot, sunny day, and he was tired of

playing hide and 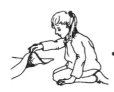. He took off his

s and sat down to read his . He

put his against the trunk of a big

 tree. The big could feel that

the boy was hot and tired, and she spread

her leaves so the sun could not shine on the

boy. The boy fell asleep. While he was

sleeping, some parts of his body began to

complain.

The said to the head, "I do not

like to be the . I am tired of holding

you up, head."

The said to the , "Hold the

head up straight, . You are causing

me to bend and be uncomfortable."

The 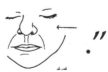 spoke to the jaw, "Please stay

closed, jaw. You are stretching me out. I do

not want to be a stretched 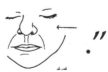."

The big 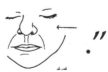 was surprised to hear all

of these grumblings. She was about to

speak when she heard the foot.

The foot said, "Why are all of you complaining? I'm the one who is almost always covered by a [sock] and a shoe. It is very

[■] and unpleasant in a [sock] and a

shoe."

The tongue spoke up, "I rarely get to

[figure] at the world. The only ones I seem to

88

get a at are doctors and dentists. It is

very  in a mouth, too."

The 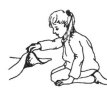 had heard enough. She said to

the body parts, "Why don't you trade

places? 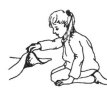 a new spot. Then maybe you

will be happier." The body parts thought

this was a great idea and agreed to do so.

The tongue tried to be the 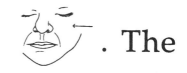 . The

 tried to be the foot. The foot tried to

be the . The  tried to be the

 . The tried to be the tongue.

When they finished switching places, they

asked the , "Well, what do you

think?"

"I think you like a ridiculous

mess," said the . "Besides, you have

ruined the poor boy's body. He can't lick

with a or sit up straight with a

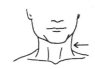 or walk on a 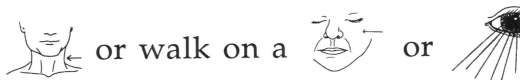 or 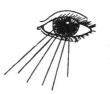 nice

with a tongue on his face."

The body parts switched to their

original places, feeling rather foolish.

91

The boy woke up and felt quite stiff and confused. He wondered what he had been dreaming about. He lifted his and began reading again.

92

Soup Thieves

Target Sound: word-final /p/   **Target Pattern:** postvocalic singletons (voiceless stops)

Target Words

	Cycle 1		Later Cycles
Pop (10)	Tip (8)	peep (13)	
soup (10)	pup (2)	sleep (1)	
cup (7)	nap (3)	lip (2)	
	shop (2)		

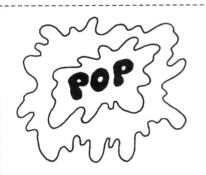

Pop

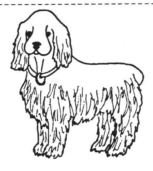

Tip

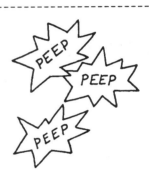

peep

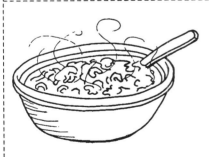

soup

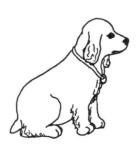

pup

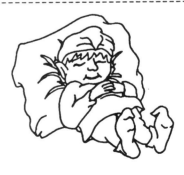

sleep

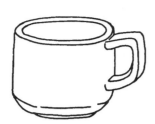

cup

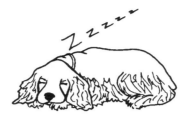

nap

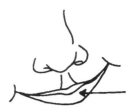

lip

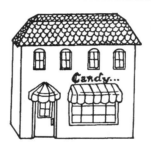

shop

94

Soup Thieves

One day the 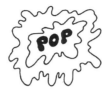 family decided to

make some 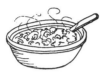 for lunch. Mr.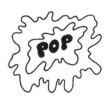

cooked the 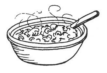 for a long time. When

he put it into a , it was too hot to eat.

Mrs. 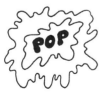 had an idea. She said, "Let's

go see the new in town, and when

95

we come back we can eat our of

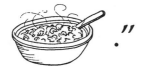 ."

So Mr. and Mrs. 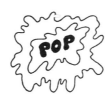 went to the new

 . They left their dog, , at

home. was no longer a little .

He liked to 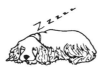 all day. was

having a nice 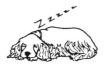 when he heard a

96

sound: " 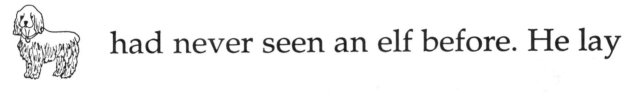 - ." opened

one eye slowly. He saw three elves climbing

up the table legs to get a [cup] of [bowl].

had never seen an elf before. He lay

very quietly and watched the elves with

one eye.

The elves began to play games and to

sing funny songs. They used a spoon to

make a slide into the . They sang:

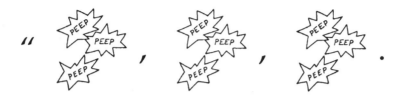

We do not like to 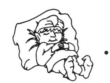 .

We play all day,

and then we say,

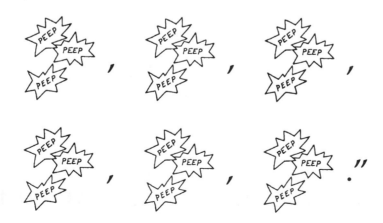

98

Mrs. 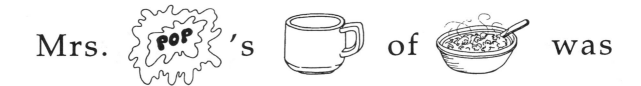's 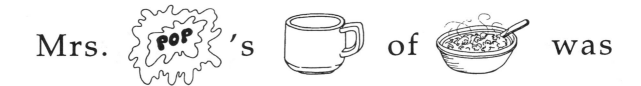 of 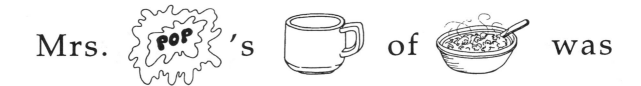 was

spilling all over the table as they jumped in

it. The elves began to get hungry, so they

leaned over the 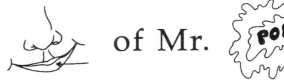 of Mr. 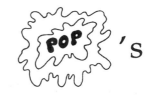's

 and took several big sips.

just watched these funny little people having

a great time.

Suddenly the elves stopped. Quick as a

wink, they slid off the of the

and down the legs of the table and disap-

peared through a crack in the wall just as

Mr. and Mrs. 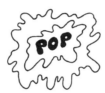 came home.

"I hope my of 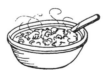 is not

hot," said Mrs. 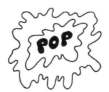 as she hung up her

coat.

"Oh, no," said Mr. 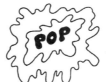. "The table is

a mess. The 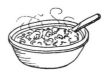 is all over it. I'll bet

 bumped the table and spilled our

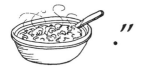 ."

"Oh ," said Mr. 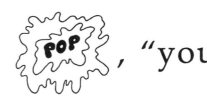 , "you

need to be more careful when you walk.

You spilled our 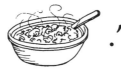 ."

101

Poor 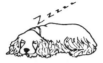 . He could not tell them his

story. He just closed his eyes to take a

, and he hoped that he would never

hear that " PEEP PEEP PEEP - PEEP PEEP PEEP " sound again.

Help for Mike

Target Sound: word-final /k/   **Target Pattern:** velars

Target Words

Cycle 1   *Later Cycles*

Mike (11)   book (2)   bike (3)   rake (6)   week (2)   backpack (3)

Rick (5)   hike (2)   lake (3)   block (2)

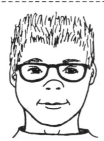

Mike

© 1993 Thinking Publications
Phonobuilding—"Help for Mike"

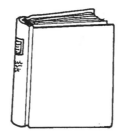

book

© 1993 Thinking Publications
Phonobuilding—"Help for Mike"

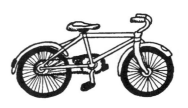

bike

© 1993 Thinking Publications
Phonobuilding—"Help for Mike"

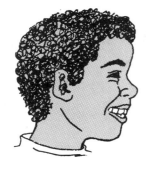

Rick

© 1993 Thinking Publications
Phonobuilding—"Help for Mike"

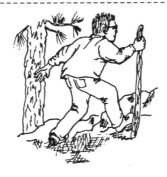

hike

© 1993 Thinking Publications
Phonobuilding—"Help for Mike"

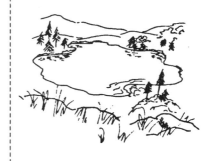

lake

© 1993 Thinking Publications
Phonobuilding—"Help for Mike"

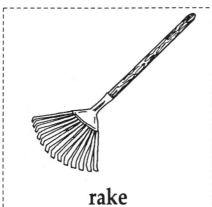

rake

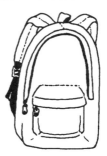

week

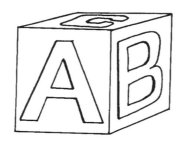

backpack

block

Help for Mike

 dropped his s and his

 on the table as he called to his

mother. "Hi Mom! I'm home!" She walked

into the kitchen and said hello. "I'm going

to go on a 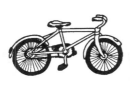  by the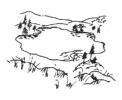

tomorrow," said .

's mother looked at him. "You

know you have to 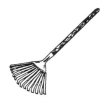 the leaves first.

That is your chore for the 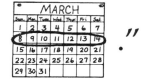 ."

 had forgotten about 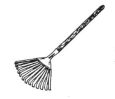ing

the leaves. He quickly reached to pick up

his s and his 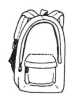. He put them

away and raced into the garage to find a

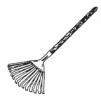 and a can to put the leaves in.

 began 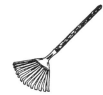 ing the leaves, but

each time he made a pile, the wind blew

and scattered the leaves across the lawn

and down the .

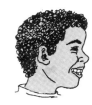 came by to ask about the

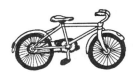 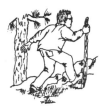 . said, "I don't

think I'll be able to go. I can't get these

leaves ed up. This is my chore for

the 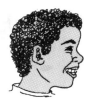 ."

 said, "I'll help. I'll the

wind while you put the leaves into the

can."

With the help of 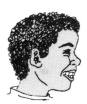, the job was

soon finished. was very happy.

The next day, set out on his

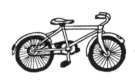 with 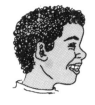 and his dad. They

rode to the 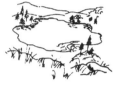 . Each boy carried a

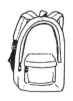 with a sack lunch inside. It was fun

to watch the leaves blow across the grass

and into the 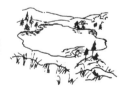 . "I wonder who has to

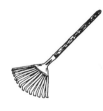 all these leaves," said .

and 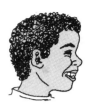 both laughed at the

thought.

Cookies for the King

Target Sounds: word-initial /k/

Target Pattern: velars (for fronting)

Target Words

Cycle 1

cow (9) cup (1) cap (4)

Later Cycles

corn (1) candy (2) king (12)

cane (2) come (2) cookie (17)

cake (1)

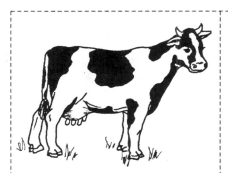

cow

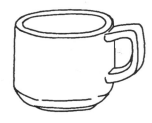

cup

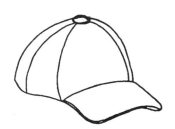

cap

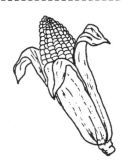

corn

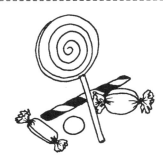

candy

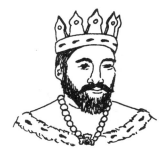

king

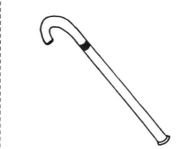

cane

© 1993 Thinking Publications
Phonobuilding—"Cookies for the King"

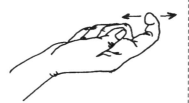

come

© 1993 Thinking Publications
Phonobuilding—"Cookies for the King"

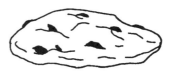

cookie

© 1993 Thinking Publications
Phonobuilding—"Cookies for the King"

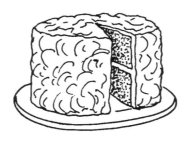

cake

© 1993 Thinking Publications
Phonobuilding—"Cookies for the King"

Cookies for the King

Once upon a time, there was a

who carried a . He was a very good

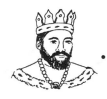 . One day he wanted a 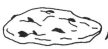 , so he

went to the kitchen to talk to the cook. The

cook said, "There is not even one 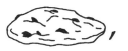 ,

because this morning I found the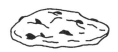

jar smashed on the floor and every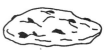

was gone."

The was sad. The cook said, "We

have some birthday ." But the

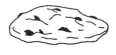 said, "No, thank you. I only want a

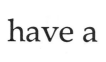 today." Then the cook said, "Well, we

have a 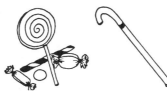 and some 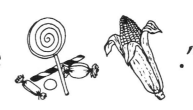."

But the said, "No, thank you. I only

want a 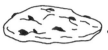." The 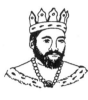 took a

of juice and went outside to try to find out

who stole the s and broke the

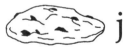 jar.

The found some footprints outside

the kitchen that looked like those of a

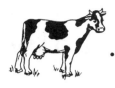. Next to the footprints was a red

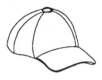. The picked up the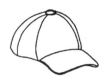

and followed the footprints across the field

to the farm down the road. There he met a

little, black and white 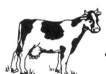. The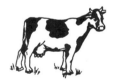

had some 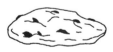 crumbs on her face, and

she had a 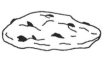 hidden in the hay.

"I see you found my red 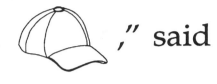," said

the  to the 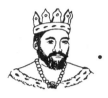.

The was angry. He asked the

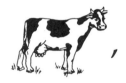, "Why did you steal my 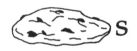s

and break my 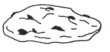 jar?"

The 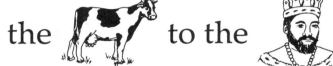 said, "I'm sorry, but I was so

hungry. The farmer gives me only hay, and

sometimes I like a 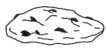. I can smell the

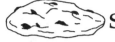s when your cook is baking them.

Last night I was taking a 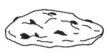 when the

jar fell on the floor and broke."

The 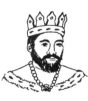 handed the to the

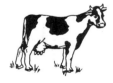 and said, "Next time, 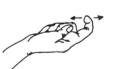 to the

kitchen when the cook is there, and he will

give you a 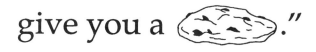."

The 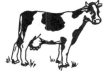 was much happier. The

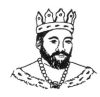 was sure the 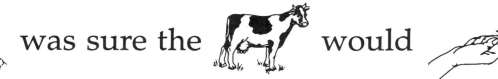 would 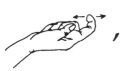,

so he went home and asked the cook to

bake lots of 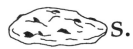s.

Come Follow Me

Target Sound: word-initial /k/

Target Pattern: velars (for fronting)

Target Words

Cycle 1

car (3)   cap (1)   come (6)

Later Cycles

carry (2)	kids (6)	country (1)
cool (2)	call (3)	can (4)
canary (12)		

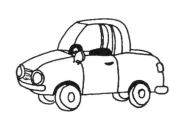

car

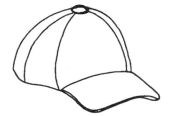

cap

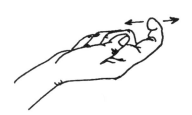

come

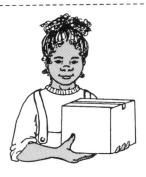

carry

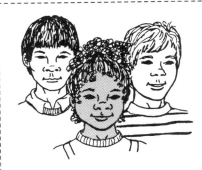

kids

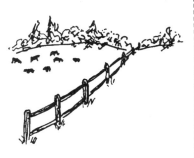

country

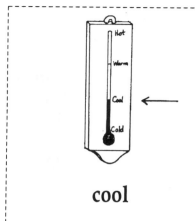

cool

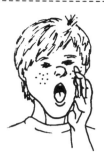

call

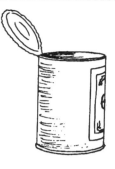

can

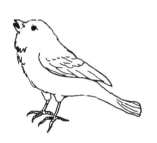

canary

Come Follow Me

Once upon a time, there were three 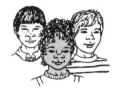 who wanted to go for a walk. It

was summertime, but the day was very

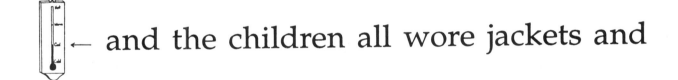 ← and the children all wore jackets and

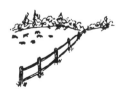s. They left the small cottage where

they lived in the 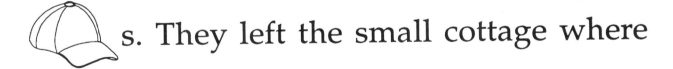 and began to

journey down a path in front of their

cottage. The 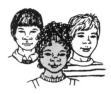 had not gone far

when they saw a yellow and blue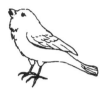

flying among the trees.

" 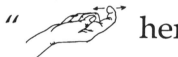 here, !" they ed.

" 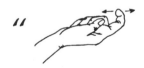 here, 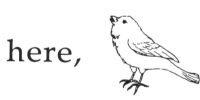 !" echoed back

from the hills.

To the surprise of the 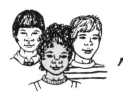 , the

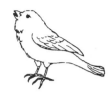 did 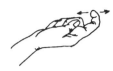 to them. He landed on a

branch above their heads and began to sing:

" 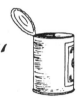 you follow me,

" you follow me,

" 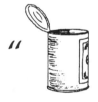 you follow me wherever I go?"

Then the 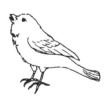 flew off. The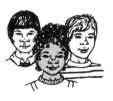

spread their arms like wings and ran down

the path, following the 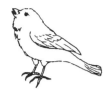 . Soon their

feet were lifted from the ground and the

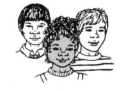 were flying, just like the 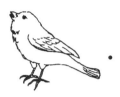 .

They flew over their cottage and over

their 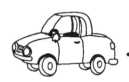 . They enjoyed the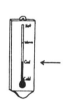

breeze on their faces. They enjoyed flying

through the air behind the 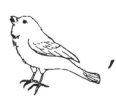 , who

was still singing his song. They noticed

their mother as she tried to 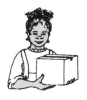 groceries

from the 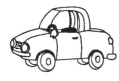 into the house.

"I think we should help those

bags," one of the 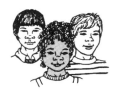 said.

They ed to the and said,

" 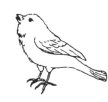 , please you help us

land? We need to stop flying."

127

The 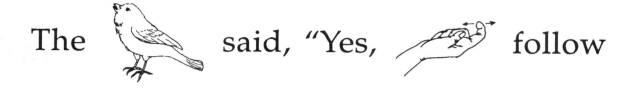 said, "Yes, follow

me."

Quickly, they headed down toward the

cottage. They yelled, "We're ing

down!" As they came close to the ground,

they put their feet down and made won-

derful landings.

"Thank you," they ed to their new

friend. " 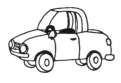 back another day." Then

they ran to the to help their mother

and to tell her about their flying adventure.

Two Ants Travel

Target Words

Cycle 1			*Later Cycles*		
Tim (8)	Tom (5)	two (3)	tiny (4)	tired (4)	together (2)
tall (4)	Tam (3)	time (7)			
	toys (3)				

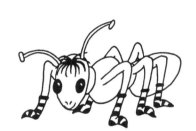

Tim

© 1993 Thinking Publications
Phonobuilding—"Two Ants Travel"

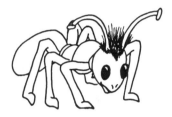

Tom

© 1993 Thinking Publications
Phonobuilding—"Two Ants Travel"

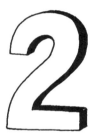

two

© 1993 Thinking Publications
Phonobuilding—"Two Ants Travel"

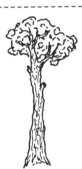

tall

© 1993 Thinking Publications
Phonobuilding—"Two Ants Travel"

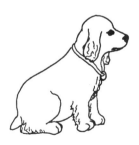

Tam

© 1993 Thinking Publications
Phonobuilding—"Two Ants Travel"

time

© 1993 Thinking Publications
Phonobuilding—"Two Ants Travel"

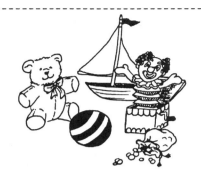

toys

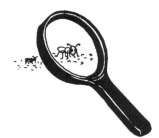

tiny

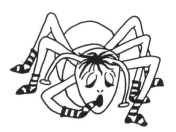

tired

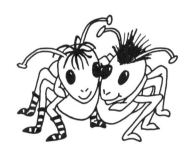

together

Two Ants Travel

Once upon a , there were

ants who decided to see the world. Their

names were and 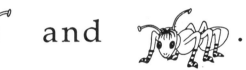 . Of

course, they were brothers. The 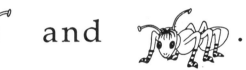 ants

packed pieces of food and their

in their packs and strapped them to

their backs. Then they walked out of their

anthill and looked around.

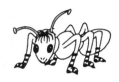 had a map. He looked at his

map. To the ants, this map looked very large,

but it was only a map of their neighborhood.

"Let's go west," said 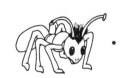 .

So they folded their map and set off.

They saw a very 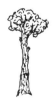 tree ahead of

them.

"Let's try to reach the tree by lunch

 and then we can stop to eat and

play with our 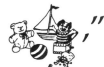," said 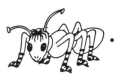.

The ants started to walk quickly, but as

the morning passed, they had to slow

down. They were so 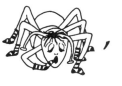, and the

tree still seemed so far away.

"Let's sing a song to make the

135

pass," said 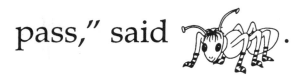.

Their cheery little song did help to make

the pass, but the ants were too

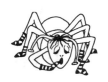 to reach the 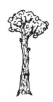 tree for lunch.

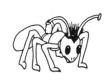 and 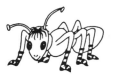 found some 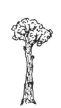 grass

and sat down. They ate their lunch quickly

and then lay down to rest. They were too

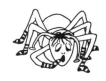 to play with their 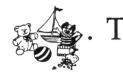. The

ants were so 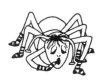 they fell asleep. When

they awoke, it was dark and to go

home. 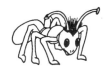 said, "We'd better stick

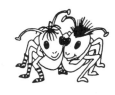. We are a long way from home."

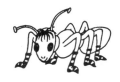 heard a noise. A pup named

 was coming down the sidewalk.

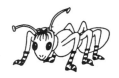 had an idea. "Hang on to my

legs," he said.

The ants joined 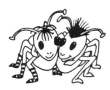, leg to leg. As

 approached, 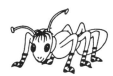 grabbed onto

her fur, and carried them all the

way home in a very short .

When they reached their anthill, the

ants let go of 's fur and dropped off.

"That was a better way to travel," said

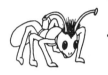 . "The next we want to see

the world, let's just find a pup to take us

where we want to go, and then we'll find

another pup to bring us back home."

The **2** ants agreed.

Necktie Finds a New Home

Target Sound: word-initial /n/   **Target Pattern:** alveolars

Target Words

Cycle 1

no (5)   night (2)   knife (3)

noise (2)   knob (4)

Later Cycles

neck(2)   necklace (9)   neighbor (2)

necktie (11)   needle (10)

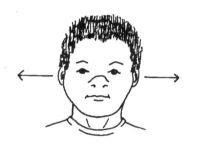

no

© 1993 Thinking Publications
Phonobuilding—"Necktie Finds a New Home"

night

© 1993 Thinking Publications
Phonobuilding—"Necktie Finds a New Home"

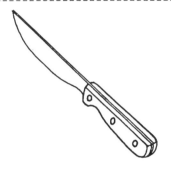

knife

© 1993 Thinking Publications
Phonobuilding—"Necktie Finds a New Home"

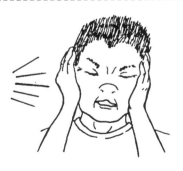

noise

© 1993 Thinking Publications
Phonobuilding—"Necktie Finds a New Home"

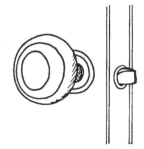

knob

© 1993 Thinking Publications
Phonobuilding—"Necktie Finds a New Home"

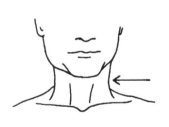

neck

© 1993 Thinking Publications
Phonobuilding—"Necktie Finds a New Home"

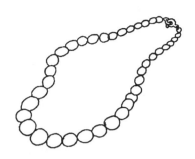

necklace

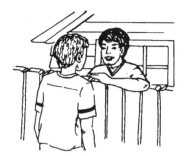

neighbor

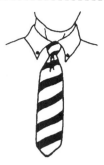

necktie

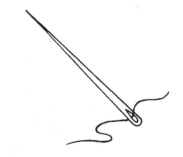

needle

Necktie Finds a New Home

Once upon a time, a neglected 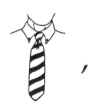,

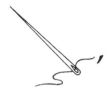, and 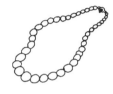 were stuck on a shelf

in the corner of a closet. They were

neglected because body ever used

them. The was 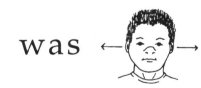 longer in

style. The 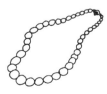 had a broken clasp. The

143

had just been forgotten.

One 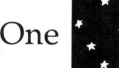, the  whispered to the

 and the 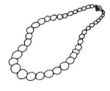 that they should go

on a journey. He was sure 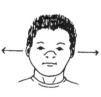 one

would miss them. His friends agreed. The

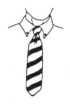 rolled to the floor, and the 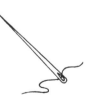 and

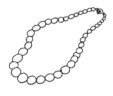 followed. They made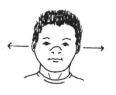

144

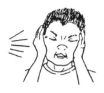 . They moved to the closet door,

which was open. They wriggled out the

door and across the room. It was very dark,

for it was  time, and the family who

lived in the house was sleeping.

The three friends crept down the stairs.

They couldn't get outside. The door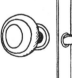

wouldn't turn because the front door was

locked. "We need a key," said the .

"Key, where are you?" called the 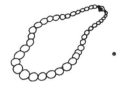 .

"Over here, on the counter by the 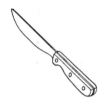 ," called the key. "If we wrap the

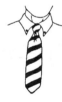 around the door , I can climb up

and unlock the door," said the key.

"Good idea," said the 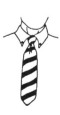 as he wrapped himself around the door 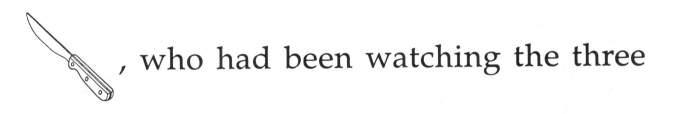.

Soon the door turned. The door

was unlocked and opened.

"Where are you going?" asked the

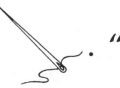, who had been watching the three

friends.

"On a journey," said the . "We'll

147

tell you about it when we return."

"Have fun," said the 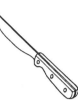 and the key.

Once they were outside, the  said,

"Let's go this way. I do not want to get near

that 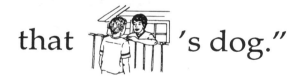's dog."

The three friends could hear the 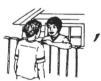's

dog barking and making a lot of 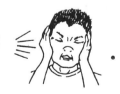.

They moved down the street. There was

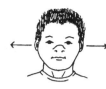 one outside. They wandered into a

field, where the 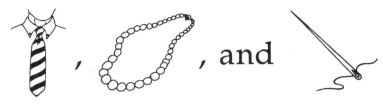, and

were introduced to a bird and a chipmunk.

"I would love to put you around my

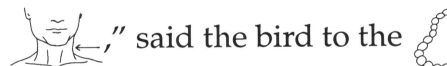," said the bird to the 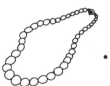.

"I would love to put *you* around my

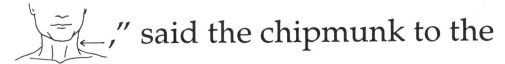," said the chipmunk to the 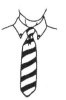.

The 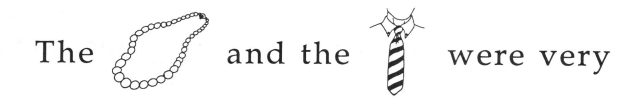 and the were very

happy to be worn again.

The bird looked at the and

asked, "May I use you to sew my nest

together? It keeps coming apart."

"I would love to sew again," said the

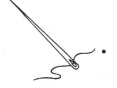

The  , the , and the

never returned home, for they had found a

new home where they were needed.

Spoon and the Funny Spice

Target Sound: word-initial /s/ blends—/sp/

Target Pattern: /s/ clusters
(for stridency and consonant clusters)

Target Words

Cycle 1

sparks (4) Spade (11) spice (9)

space (1) speak (2) spot (4)

Spoon (15)

Later Cycles

spaceship (6)

spinning (9)

speedy (1)

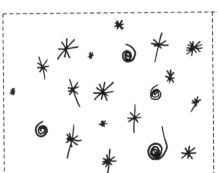

sparks

© 1993 Thinking Publications
Phonobuilding—"Spoon and the Funny Spice"

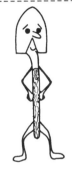

Spade

© 1993 Thinking Publications
Phonobuilding—"Spoon and the Funny Spice"

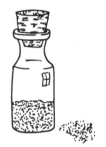

spice

© 1993 Thinking Publications
Phonobuilding—"Spoon and the Funny Spice"

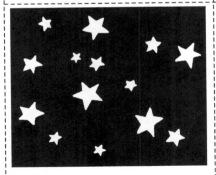

space

© 1993 Thinking Publications
Phonobuilding—"Spoon and the Funny Spice"

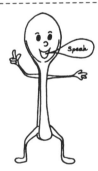

speak

© 1993 Thinking Publications
Phonobuilding—"Spoon and the Funny Spice"

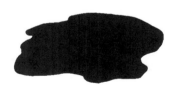

spot

© 1993 Thinking Publications
Phonobuilding—"Spoon and the Funny Spice"

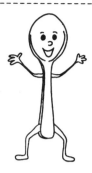

Spoon

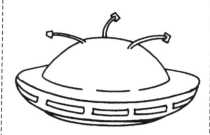

spaceship

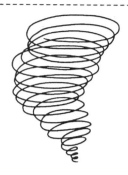

spinning

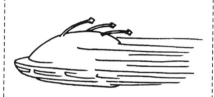

speedy

Spoon and the Funny Spice

 was standing on a special 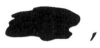,

looking off into 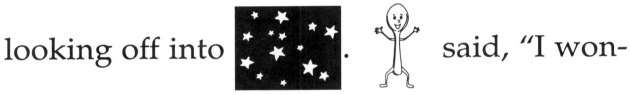. said, "I won-

der if I should to  about the

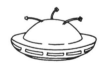 I saw last night. It landed on this

very 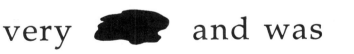 and was 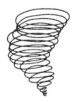 around and

around. There were everywhere."

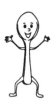 spoke in a loud voice: " 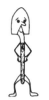 , I

have to 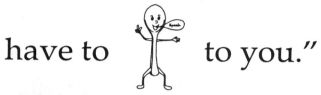 to you."

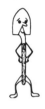 walked over to . "Hi, ,"

he said. "Why are you 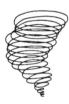 around?"

"I'm  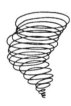 just like the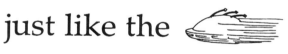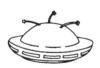

I saw last night," said .

"A 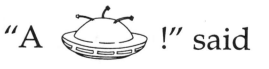 !" said 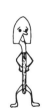 .

"Yes, a 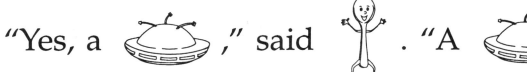," said . "A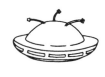

landed on this very ▬▬ . I saw it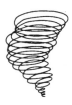

around and around. There were two crea-

tures on the . They gave me this jar

of ."

"Maybe that is not ," said 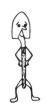 .

Slowly, 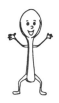 opened the jar of .

"It smells like cinnamon," said 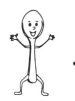 .

Suddenly, 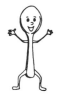 started around

and around. 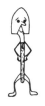 took the jar of

from . He smelled the .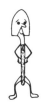

started 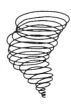 around and around just

like 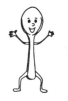 .

"I want to stop 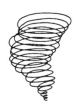 ," said 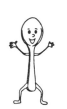 .

"I want to stop 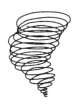," said 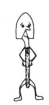.

 dropped the jar of on the

ground. flew up into the air. There

were many, many 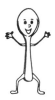.

Then 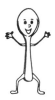 and 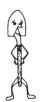 stopped 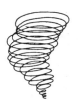.

They looked for the bottle of . It had

disappeared with the .

"I don't think that was cinnamon,"

said 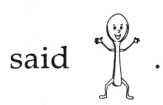 .

"That was very funny 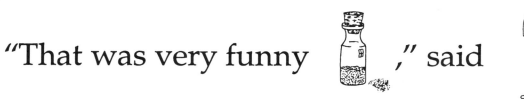," said 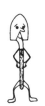 .

I think that we should go away from this

funny so we don't get any more bot-

tles of funny 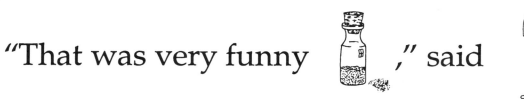."

Wishing on a Star

Target Sound: word-initial /s/ blends—/st/

Target Pattern: /s/ clusters
(for stridency and consonant clusters)

Target Words

Cycle 1

stone (12)	stem (2)	store (1)
star (7)	storm (2)	steps (3)
stamp (2)	stop (4)	stand (2)

Later Cycles

station (3)

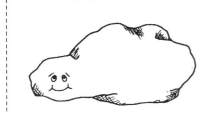

stone

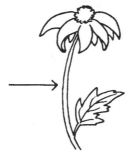

stem

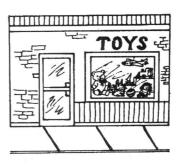

store

star

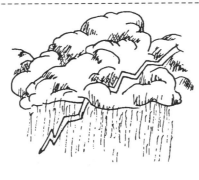

storm

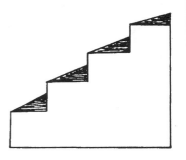

steps

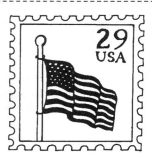

stamp

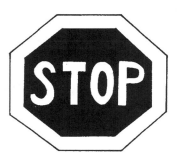

stop

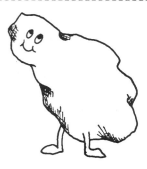

stand

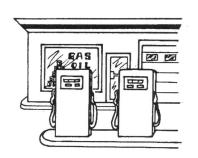

station

Wishing on a Star

Once upon a time, there was a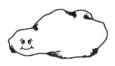

as small as a who wanted to be a

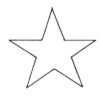 . He could not STOP looking at

the sky and wishing he could find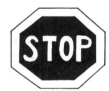

to take him to the sky. He tried to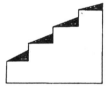

on his 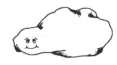 legs, but he could not even

reach the top of a flower →. The flower

bowed its → and laughed at the poor

little 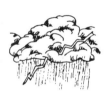.

One day, a 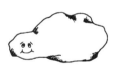 came. There were

very strong winds. The 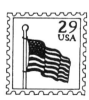 was blown

about like a postage ... He passed a

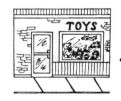. He rolled down some 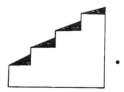.

He finally landed at a train 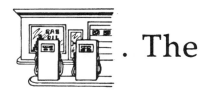. The

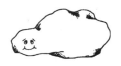 rolled onto a train just as it was

pulling out of the 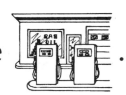.

The train traveled along the tracks. The

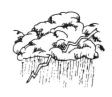 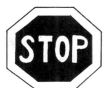ped and the sun returned to

the sky. At the first train 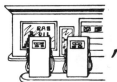, the train

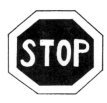ped and the 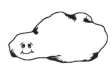 rolled down

some . It was nighttime, and there

were many 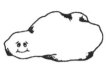s in the sky. The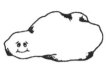

decided to make a wish. He tried to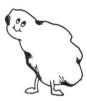

up to make his wish. He wanted the 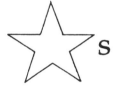s

to hear him. The 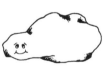 said, "I wish I

could 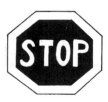 being a 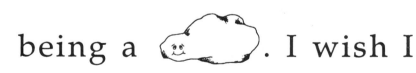. I wish I

could be a very bright 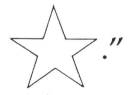."

Suddenly, there was a flash of light and

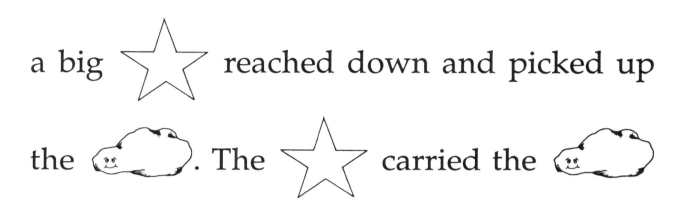

a big ⭐ reached down and picked up

the ☁. The ⭐ carried the ☁

to the sky and placed him in a very special

spot.

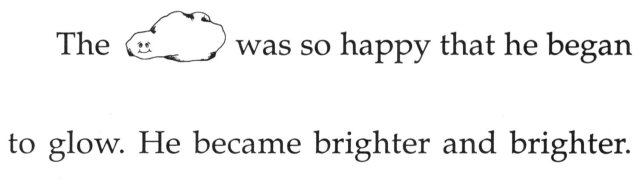

The ☁ was so happy that he began

to glow. He became brighter and brighter.

Soon he looked just like a ⭐.

Skip Dreams

Target Sound: word-initial /s/ blends—/sk/

Target Pattern: /s/ clusters
(for stridency and consonant clusters)

Target Words

Cycle 1

Skip (14)   sky (7)   ski (3)

school (2)   scoop (4)

Later Cycles

scuba (4)   skier (3)   skeleton (4)

scanning (2)   scary (1)

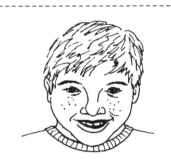

Skip

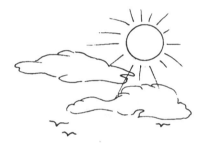

sky

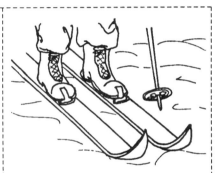

ski

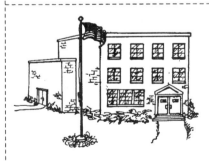

school

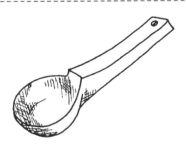

scoop

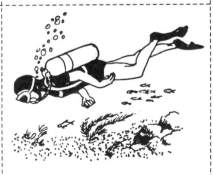

scuba

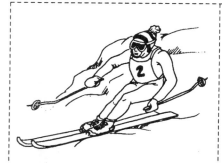

skier

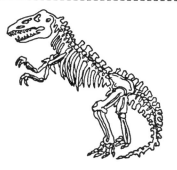

skeleton

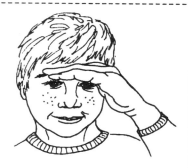

scanning

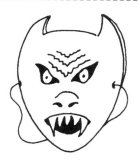

scary

Skip Dreams

 was looking at the 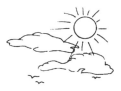 while

he was eating two 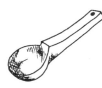s of ice cream.

The 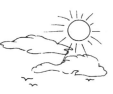 was full of clouds. Some of

them looked like 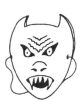 monsters. Others

looked like 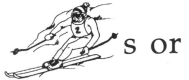s or 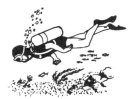 divers.

The clouds over the 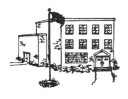 looked like

© 1993 Thinking Publications

dinosaur 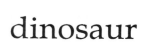 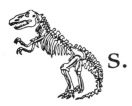 s.

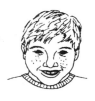 was so busy 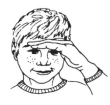 the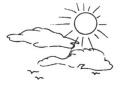

that he forgot about his ice cream. The top

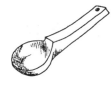 fell to the ground. quickly

ate the other 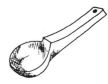 of ice cream. Then he

lay down in the grass.

The clouds began to move across the

172

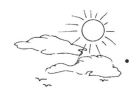 became very sleepy. He fell

asleep and began to dream that he was a

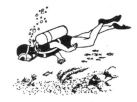 diver diving into the sea to rescue

a lost treasure. Some of 's friends

were also 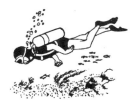 divers. They were just

about to 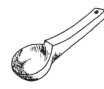 up the treasure when . . .

WHOOSH! 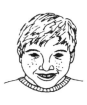 was 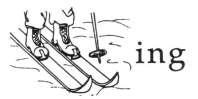ing

down a mountain covered with snow. The

other 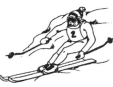s were trying to catch 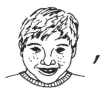,

but he was 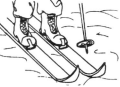ing too fast for them.

Suddenly, 's 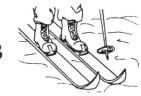s slipped on

some ice. was rolling down the

mountain toward a tree when . . .

WHOOSH! 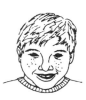 was on an expedition

looking for dinosaur s. He was the

174

leader of the expedition. and some

of the students from his 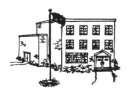 were dig-

ging in the dirt. They saw a dinosaur

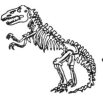 . Suddenly, the 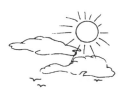 turned gray

and there was a clap of thunder. Rain began

to fall. . . .

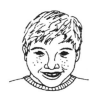 awoke from his nap on the grass.

Real raindrops were falling on his cheeks.

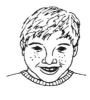 looked at the 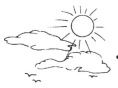. His cloud

figures were gone. 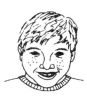 ran home,

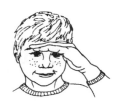 the 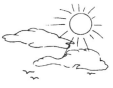 and thinking about his

adventures as a 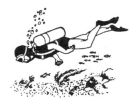 diver, 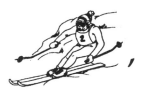,

and the leader of the dinosaur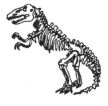

expedition.

Pups' Vacation Planning

Target Sound: word-final stop-plus /s/

Target Pattern: /s/ clusters
(for stridency, consonant clusters, and plurals)

Target Words

	Cycle 1		*Later Cycles*
pups (6)	cups (2)	books (4)	backpacks (2)
boats (5)	nights (2)	nuts (2)	
lakes (4)	shops (4)	bikes (5)	

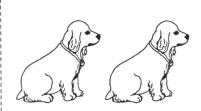

pups

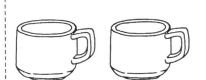

cups

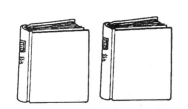

books

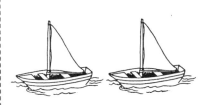

boats

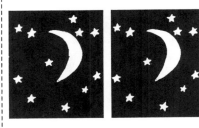

nights

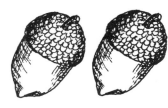

nuts

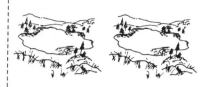

lakes

shops

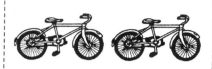

bikes

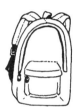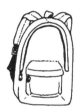

backpacks

Pups' Vacation Planning

Once upon a time, some 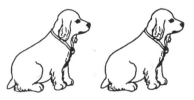 were looking through some 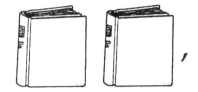, trying to find a good vacation site. The 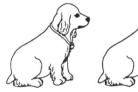 looked and looked. They looked for several  at the 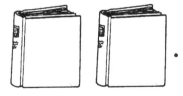. Then they found more and

179

looked for several weeks. They could not

make a decision.

Finally, they decided that a trip to a

lake would be fun. So the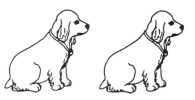

read about big 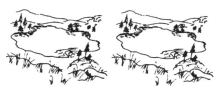 and small

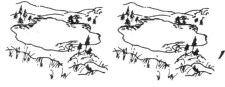 , about 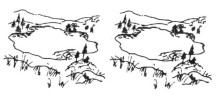 that

were close and 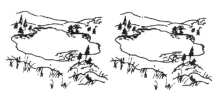 that were far

away. Their vacation was only for two

180

weeks, so they chose a close lake that was

big enough for all of the different kinds of

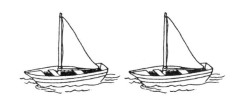 that they wanted to ride.

The 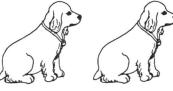 wanted to try

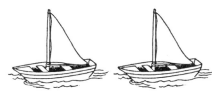 with motors,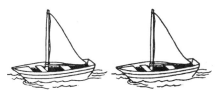

with oars, and 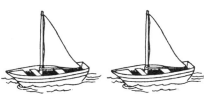 with sails.

The 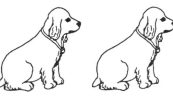 also wanted to ride

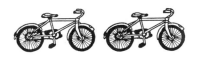 and visit   . The

vacation site chosen seemed to have trails

for 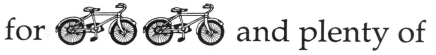 and plenty of .

The 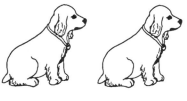 decided to travel

lightly. They each filled one backpack

with supplies. The two 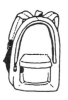 would

make traveling easy.

One day, they loaded their car with

their 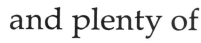 and their 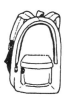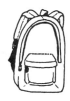 and they set off for their vacation at the lake.

After driving for several hours they

were thirsty, so they stopped for some

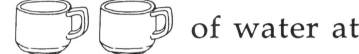 of water at a rest stop. After

drinking several 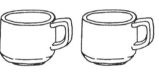 and stretching

their legs, they continued their journey.

Soon they saw the sparkling blue lake,

the trails for their 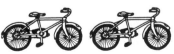, and the

183

attractive little .

They had a wonderful vacation, visit-

ing , riding 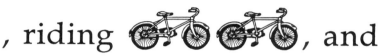, and

driving 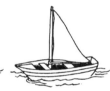. They were just

 about this vacation site. They

were so about it that they decided

to go there every year so they would not

184

have to spend so many

looking at vacation 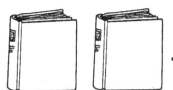 .

Playmates for Lynn

Target Sound: word-initial /l/

Target Pattern: liquids

Target Words

Cycle 1

Lynn (17)	leg (2)	land (2)
lake (6)	line (2)	log (4)
look (7)	lay (2)	

Later Cycles

lemon (5)

lady (2)

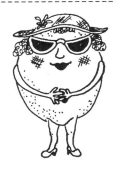

Lynn

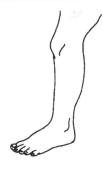

leg

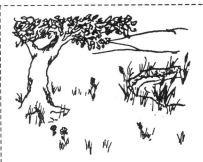

land

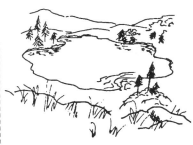

lake

line

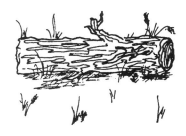

log

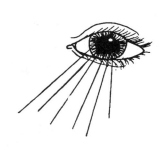

look

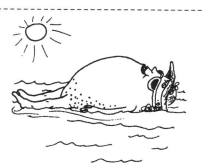

lay

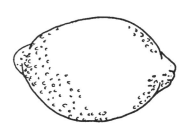

lemon

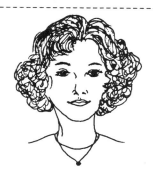

lady

Playmates for Lynn

Once upon a time, there was a

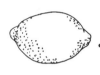. Her name was 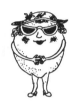. 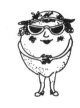 loved

to roll down the hill like a 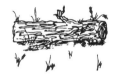 and fall

into the 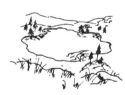. She would then float

along the top of the water looking for

playmates.

© 1993 Thinking Publications

One day when 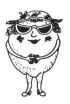 was 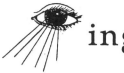ing

for some playmates, her 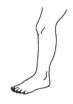 became

tangled in a fishing ——. The fisherman

reeled her in and laughed. He thought

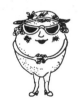 ed so funny with her cool

sunglasses and her sun hat. He asked

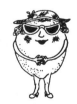, "Why are you floating in the

water?"

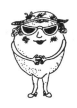 said, "I'm 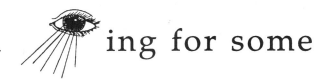ing for some

playmates."

The fisherman untangled her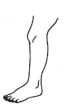

from the —————— and said, "Who would play

with a 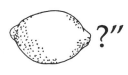?"

Then he laughed and tossed her back

into the 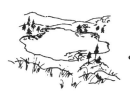. Poor 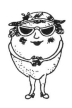. She was not finding any friends.

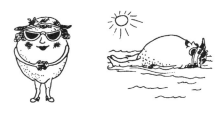 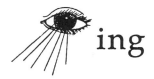 on her back 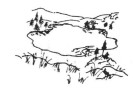 ing

into the sun and continued to float on the

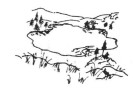 like a 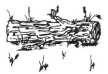. She found some

fish. She tried to swim down to the

bottom of the 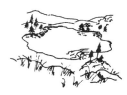 like the fish, but

she could not.

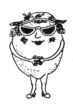 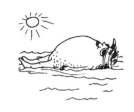 back down and

continued to float. She found some boats.

She went up to the boats and said, "Hi!"

But they just ed away and sped

across the 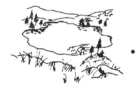 .

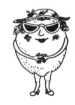 saw a green frog. She said hello

to the frog. The frog said "Ribbit!" and

193

hopped off his 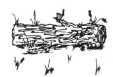 , splashing poor

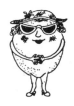 and almost upsetting her hat and

sunglasses.

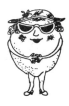 ed up at the warm sun.

"You are yellow just like me," she said. "Will

you play with me?" The sun did not answer,

but sent strong rays down to warm 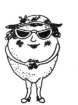 .

At last 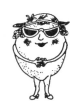 stopped floating. She

stood up and walked onto the 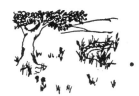 .

There were many trees on the 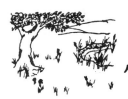 , and

they looked like they were covered with

yellow balls. "Oh, ! Those are 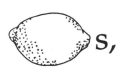s,

just like me," said 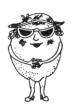 .

As she got closer, 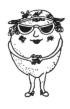 found many,

many s to play with. 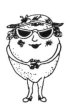 taught

the other s how to roll down the hill

like a 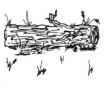 into the 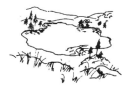. They all

had a very good time.

Santa Saves the Sleeping Baby

Target Sounds: word-initial /l/ blends   **Target Pattern:** liquids and consonant sequences

Target Words

Cycle 1	Later Cycles		
climbed (6)	sleeping (4)	flying (4)	flew (2)
glass (3)	plum (3)	sleigh (7)	blimp (5)
	blanket (4)	slippers (2)	

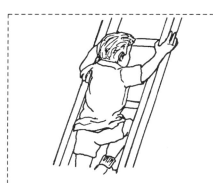

climbed

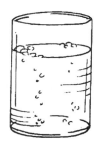

glass

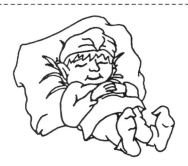

sleeping

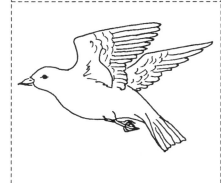

flying

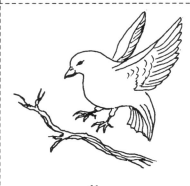

flew

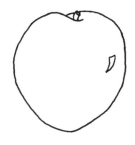

plum

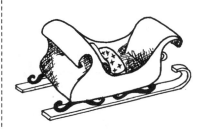

sleigh

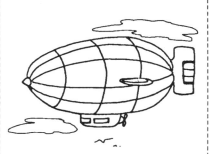

blimp

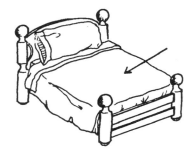

blanket

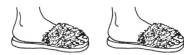

slippers

Santa Saves
the Sleeping Baby

Once upon a time, there was a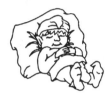

baby. She woke up from her nap, out

of bed, and crawled down the stairs and

out the door. She found a seed. She

threw it in the dirt. This funny seed

planted itself in the dirt and grew and grew

within seconds. The baby 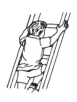 the

tree. It had grown very high. At the top of

the tree, the baby saw a purple 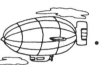. She

 into the 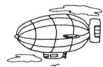, and the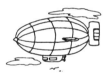

 through the sky.

The 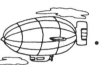 landed on the moon, and

the baby crawled out. There she saw a

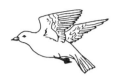 saucer. Blue people wearing

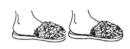 slipped from the 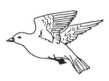 saucer to

the moon.

One blue man with 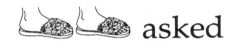 asked

the baby if she would like to ride in his

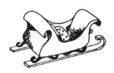. The baby aboard the blue

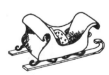. She put a blue 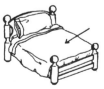 over her legs

and they to the North Pole. At the

North Pole, they met a jolly old man with a

red suit, a white beard, and es. That's

right! It was Santa Claus.

Santa Claus picked up the baby and

asked, "Does your mommy know that you

have been 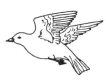 through the sky in a

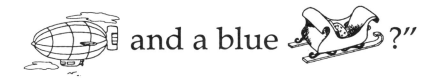 and a blue ?"

The baby just gurgled. Santa hooked

up his reindeer to his . One of his

jolly elves in and came along for the

ride. Santa drove the while the elf

held tightly to the baby wrapped in the

blue .

Soon they were at the baby's house.

Santa landed the 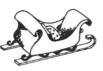 on the roof. Then

he carefully picked up the now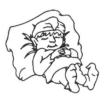

baby. He carefully down the chimney

and silently crept through the house. He

put the 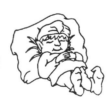 baby in her bed. Santa Claus

was soon back in his 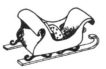 and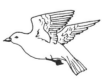

home.

204

When the 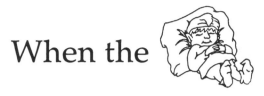 baby's mother went to

get her up from her nap, she noticed a blue

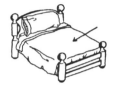 tucked around her. She wondered

where that blue had come from.

205

A Rest for Rattlesnake

Target Sound: word-initial /r/

Target Pattern: liquids

Target Words

	Cycle 1			*Later Cycles*		
rat (14)	run (3)	red (5)		road (3)	rooster (5)	replied (5)
rock (5)	rest (14)			rattlesnake (13)		robin (3)

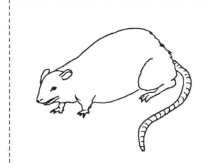

rat

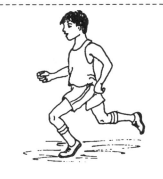

run

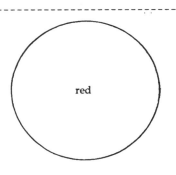

red

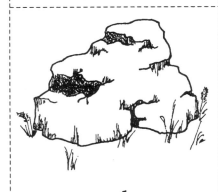

rock

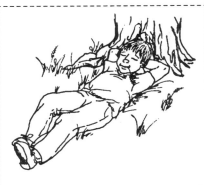

rest

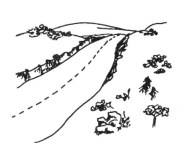

road

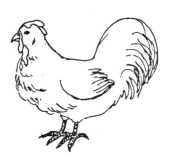

rooster

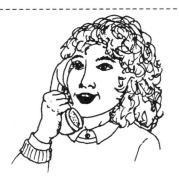

replied

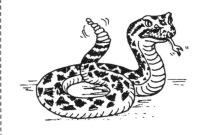

rattlesnake

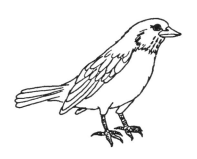

robin

A Rest for Rattlesnake

Once upon a time, in a faraway forest,

there lived a 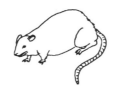 and a 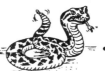. The

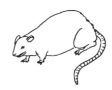 loved to tease the 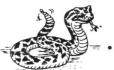. He

would close to the 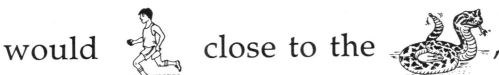, awaken

him from his , and then away.

The 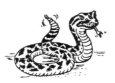 was a very sleepy rattler. He

loved to lie in the sun and 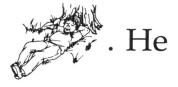 . He also

loved to eat 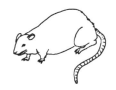 s, but he was never

able to catch this 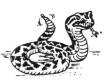 who teased him

every day.

One day, the 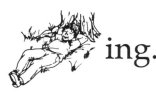 was not 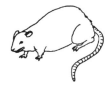 ing.

He was slithering through the tall grass

when he saw the 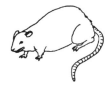 who loved to tease ing on the side of the 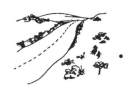.

Slowly and quietly, the 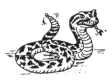 slithered

closer and closer. The 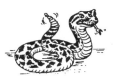 opened his

large jaws and was ready to swallow the

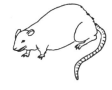 in one gulp when the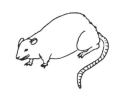

awoke from his 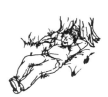 in time to

quickly away.

The 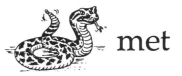 slithered off to find a

different snack. On the way, the 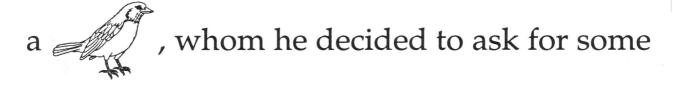 met

a 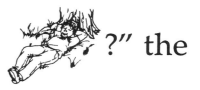 , whom he decided to ask for some

advice. "Where can I get some 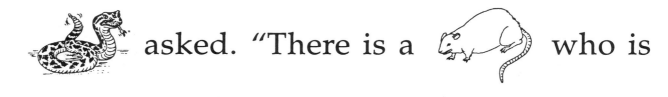 ?" the

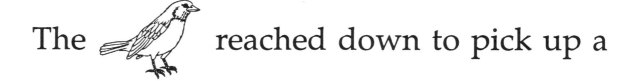 asked. "There is a who is

always bothering me."

The reached down to pick up a

worm. She ate the worm and then 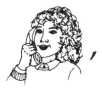,

"Why don't you 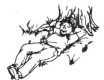 in a tree, just like

me? I don't think the 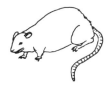 could bother

you there."

The snake , "The 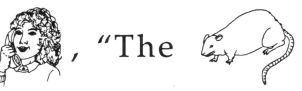 can

climb, so I cannot 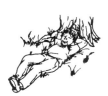 in a tree, but

thank you for your time, 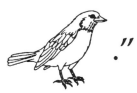."

The snake continued to slither down the

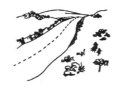. He met a . The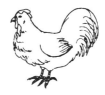

was 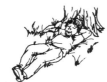ing on a roost near the barn-

yard. "Hello, ," said the 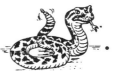. "I

was wondering if you could help me.

There is a 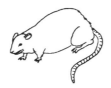 who never allows me to

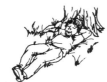. He is always bothering me. What

should I do?"

The 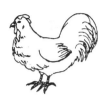, after pecking at

some corn, "Why don't you find a roost,

just like me? I don't think the 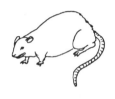 could

bother you there."

The snake , "I cannot 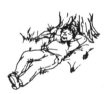 on a

roost, but thank you for your time,

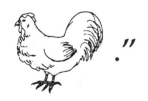."

The snake continued to slither down

the 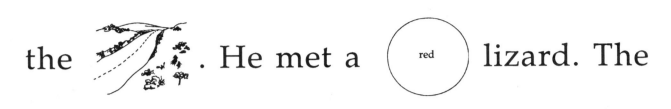 . He met a (red) lizard. The

(red) lizard was sitting by a pond catch-

ing bugs with his tongue. "Hello, (red)

lizard," said the 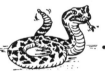 . "I was wondering

if you could help me. There is a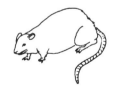

who never allows me to 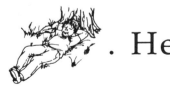 . He is

always bothering me. What should I do?"

The lizard 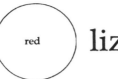, after catching

some flies, "Why don't you find a 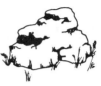 to

crawl under, just like me? The 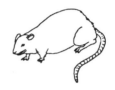 won't

think to look for you under a 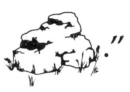."

"Under a 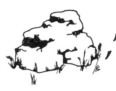," thought the 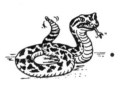.

"You think I should 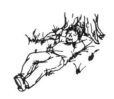 under a

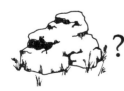? Well, I think that is a wonderful

idea. I will go 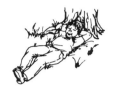 under a 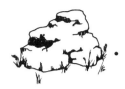 .

Goodbye, 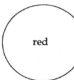 lizard, and thank you."

Fox and the Fat Fish

Target Sound: word-initial /f/   **Secondary Target Pattern:** anterior strident singletons

Target Words

	Cycle 1		*Later Cycles*
fun (2)	fox (7)	four (3)	forest (2)
fins (2)	fish (9)	find (2)	
foot (3)	fat (6)	food (3)	

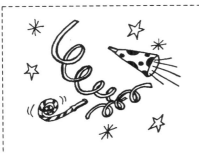

fun

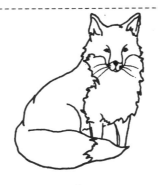

fox

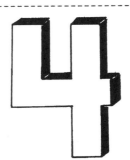

four

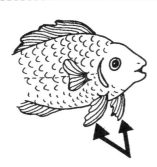

fins

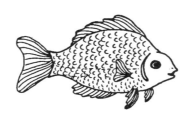

fish

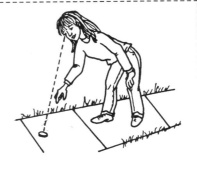

find

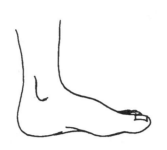

foot

© *1993 Thinking Publications*
Phonobuilding—"Fox and the Fat Fish"

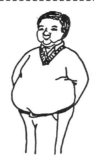

fat

© *1993 Thinking Publications*
Phonobuilding—"Fox and the Fat Fish"

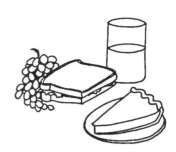

food

© *1993 Thinking Publications*
Phonobuilding—"Fox and the Fat Fish"

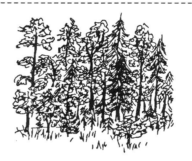

forest

© *1993 Thinking Publications*
Phonobuilding—"Fox and the Fat Fish"

Fox and the Fat Fish

Once upon a time, there was a

who sat at the edge of a pond watching

  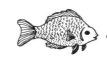 . They wriggled their

 and their bodies sparkled as they

swam around the pond. The 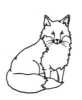 wanted

to eat the   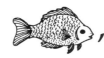 , for he was very

hungry. Each time he stuck his into

the water to grab a 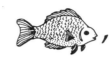, the

darted away.

"This is  teasing the ," said

the 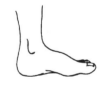. "Let's swim close to his

and then we will dart away."

The 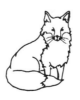 became frustrated as the

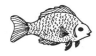 swam closer and closer but never

close enough for him to grab one of them.

One time he swiped at one of their  ,

but that 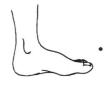 wriggled away from his

.

The walked away from the water.

He felt unhappy because he was so hungry.

"Maybe I can some 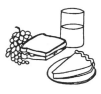 in the

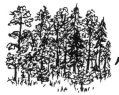," he thought. He wandered toward

the 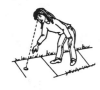. On his way, he happened to

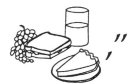 some delicious, ripe strawberries.

"Strawberries are my favorite 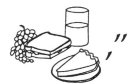,"

he said. He reached down to pluck one

berry. It was delicious. He ate strawberries

until he was full. Now the 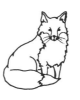 felt 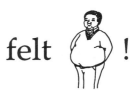 !

Then the went back to the pond

to watch the that he had

wanted to feast on earlier that day. "It is

 to watch these ," he

said. "I am glad I found some other

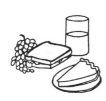 to eat."

Sam's Magnificent Scene

Target Sound: word-initial /s/   **Secondary Target Pattern:** anterior strident singletons

Target Words

Cycle 1

same (2)   some (4)   sat (2)

sea (6)   Sam (15)   sound (2)

saw (4)

Later Cycles

submarine (7)

sandwich (3)

cinnamon (2)

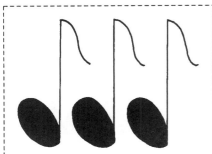

same

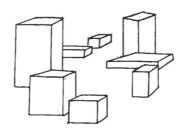

some

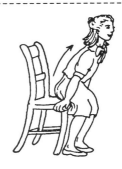

sat

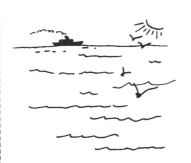

sea

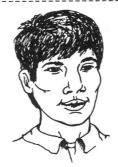

Sam

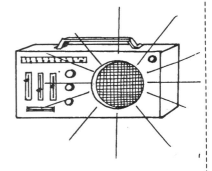

sound

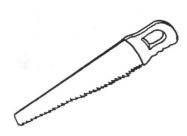

saw

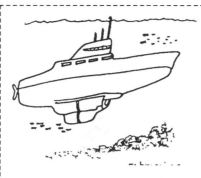

submarine

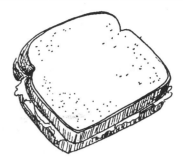

sandwich

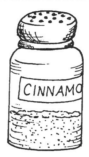

cinnamon

Sam's Magnificent Scene

Once upon a time, there was a boy

named 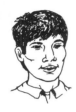 who was tired of doing the

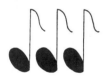 things every day. So he

down and decided to draw himself a

magnificent scene so large that he could

jump right into it.

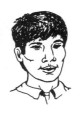 began to draw. First, he drew

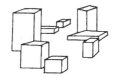 water. The water was clean and

sparkling, but it did not make a 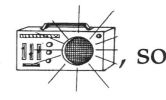, so

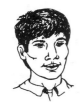 drew a waterfall. The water splashed

loudly as it cascaded down one side of

the drawing. "It seems to 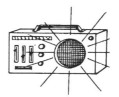 like a

symphony," thought 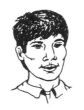 .

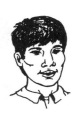

At the bottom of the waterfall,

drew a peaceful lake. On the bottom of the

lake, he drew a 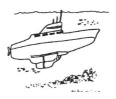 with a tall

periscope so the people in the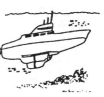

could spy on the people on the beach.

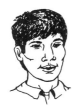 drew himself in the picture as

well. He 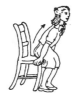 in the captain's chair of the

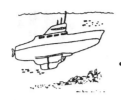 . He pulled in the periscope and

headed out to 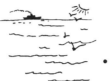 . The 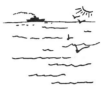 was a

large ocean. 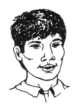 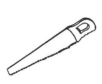 many kinds of

fish. None of them looked the 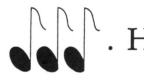 . He

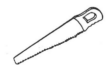 a swordfish, an octopus, and a

shark. Looking out one of the portholes,

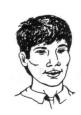 even a blue whale.

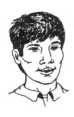 decided to go scuba diving. He

brought the 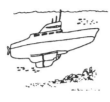 to the surface. He put

on his scuba gear and dove into the

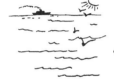. He swam slowly to the bottom of

the 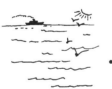. He found a boat that

appeared to have been shipwrecked long

ago.

On board the ship were some chests.

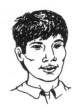 knew there would be treasure in the

chests. He drew a crane long enough to

reach down from the 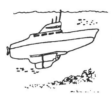 and lift the

treasure chests to the surface of the 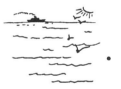 .

It was a very strong crane.

When 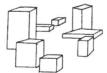 of the chests were safely

loaded onto the 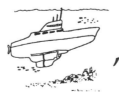 , 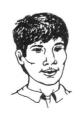 took off

234

his scuba gear and drew a tool to open

the chests. They opened easily. Inside,

  not 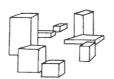 treasure, but

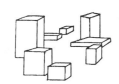 rolls. The rolls were not

soggy, so ate one, two, three

rolls. These rolls made 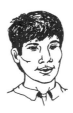 realize that

he was very hungry, so quickly he jour-

neyed back through the 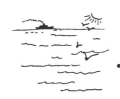 . He left

his 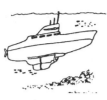 in the lake at the bottom of

the noisy waterfall.

He was just going to draw himself a

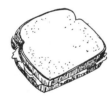 when he realized he did not want a

picture of a 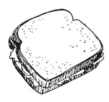. He wanted a real

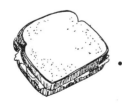. "Mom," he called. "Can I have

lunch?"

"Yes," said his mother. "What have you

been doing all morning?"

"Oh, just going here and there," said

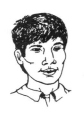 .

Fox Goes to First Grade

Target Sound: word-final /st/ blends   **Advanced Target Pattern:** complex consonant sequences
(for stridency and consonant clusters)

Target Words

Cycle 1   *Later Cycles*

first (12)	rest (4)	test (2)
forest (4)	most (2)	cast (2)
last (3)	best (5)	roast (4)
	past (3)	

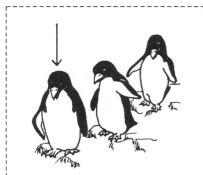

first

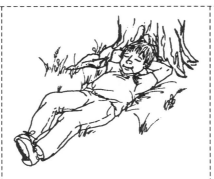

rest

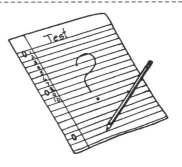

test

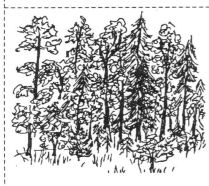

forest

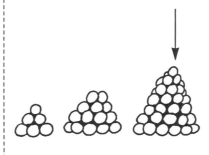

most

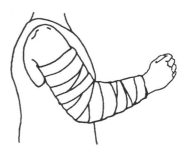

cast

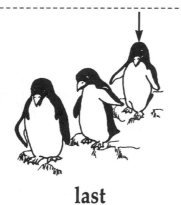

last

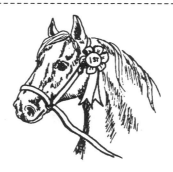

best

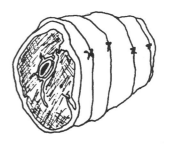

roast

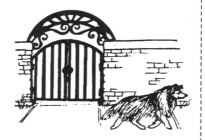

past

Fox Goes to First Grade

Once upon a time, there was a fox who

was six years old. He lived near the 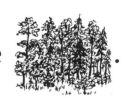.

He knew that at 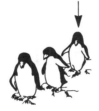 the time was com-

ing when he would have to go to school.

Now this fox just did *not* want to go to

school. He liked to play with his box of

school supplies and his new books, but he

did not like the idea of going to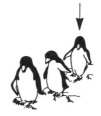

grade.

" 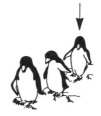 grade," he thought. "I will be

in school all day. I will need to pack my

lunch in a box. I will need to stand at the

bus stop with the other big foxes. Maybe I

will be the 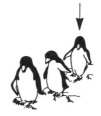 one on the bus. Maybe

242

the bus will leave without me. Maybe I will

be 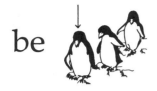 on the bus and I won't be able to

climb those big steps. Maybe I will have to

take a . I think taking a  is too

hard for me. Oh dear, this is too much for

me. I will pack some supplies in my box

and run away to the 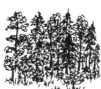 . Then I will not

have to go to grade."

Fox opened his box and packed a

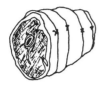

beef sandwich, cookies, juice, and

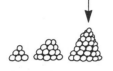

of his favorite storybooks. Then he

walked out of the house and toward the

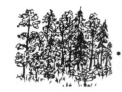

. His mother would be so worried

when she discovered that he was gone.

Along the road to the 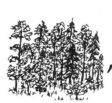, he met

some of his neighbors. "Hello," he called as

he walked 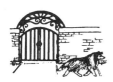 them. After walking

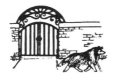 two more houses, the fox was tired.

He stopped to 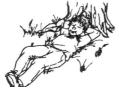. He opened his

lunch box and ate his 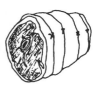 beef sand-

wich and a cookie. He drank some juice

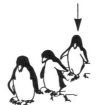. Then he looked at his books.

"I like to just look at my books, but I

wish someone were here to read these

books to me," thought the fox. After his

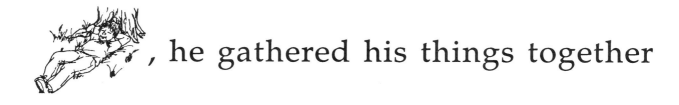, he gathered his things together

and went on his way to find someone to

read his 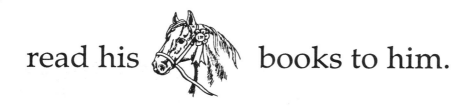 books to him.

Fox met a buzzing wasp. "Can you read

these books to me?" he asked.

"Oh, no," said the wasp, who was

making a 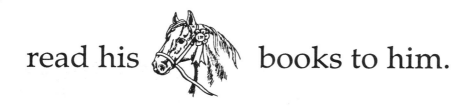. "I cannot read. I never

went to school." The wasp continued

cooking his 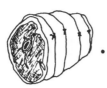.

Next the fox met a chicken with a

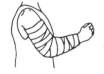. "Do you have time to read these

books to me?" he asked.

"Oh, no", said the chicken with a

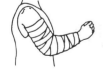. "I am a very busy chicken. I have

no time to 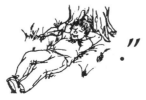."

Then the fox met a chipmunk. "Mr.

Chipmunk, can you read me a story from

one of my 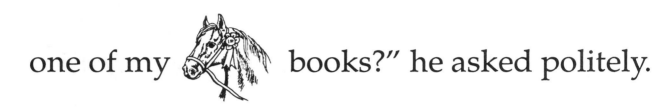 books?" he asked politely.

"No, Fox, I cannot read to you today.

But soon school will start, and when you go

to school, the 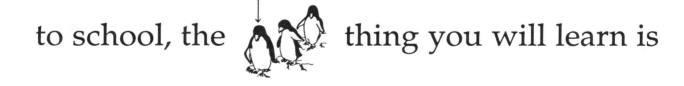 thing you will learn is

how to read those books all by yourself."

"Well," said the fox, "I'm running away

so I don't ever have to go to school. I don't

want to go to grade. Did you say

that I could learn to read in 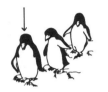 grade?"

asked the fox thoughtfully.

"Yes," said the chipmunk. "There are

many books in 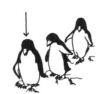 grade for all the

children to read."

"I think I had better go home and discuss

 grade with my mother," said the fox.

So off he trotted back down the road to

his house. He walked 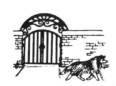 his neighbors'

houses and then came to his own. He went

inside and found his mother. "Mother, will

I learn to read books in 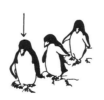 grade?"

asked the fox.

"Of course," she said. "It may take some

time, but reading is one of the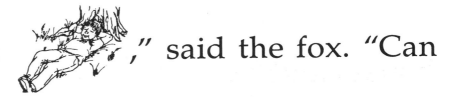

important reasons for going to school."

"I need a 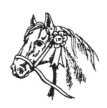," said the fox. "Can

you read my storybook to me?" he

asked.

"Yes," said his mother.

251

The next week, on the  day of

school, the fox had no trouble at the bus

stop. He had decided he would try to do

his very 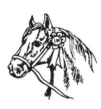 work at school. The other

foxes were very nice to him. When he

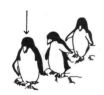 arrived at school, he saw his teacher

and his classroom. It was filled with books.

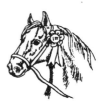

The fox decided that school was the

place he had ever seen.

Primary Level Vocabulary Sheet

word	sketch	explanation	word used in a sentence

Upper Elementary Level
Vocabulary Sheet

word	sketch	explanation	word used in a sentence

Appendix B

Levels of Narrative Development

The acquisition of narrative skills seems to follow a developmental progression, with early developing skills providing the foundation for later acquired skills. Applebee (1978) has outlined six basic types of narrative structure, followed by four additional levels of narrative development, based on Piaget's levels of cognitive development (Ault, 1977). Examples of children's narratives* are from Hedburg and Stoel-Gammon (1986).

Types of Narrative Structure

Heaps—Heaps are the earliest prenarrative structure. These are collections of unrelated ideas. Children switch topics freely with no apparent connections between the utterances. The sentences are generally simple declarations, usually in the present or present progressive tenses (Westby, 1984). Cohesive techniques are not used. "Children who tell heap stories often do not appear to recognize that the characters on each page of picture books are the same characters" (Westby, 1984, p. 115). For example a child might say:

> A dog is walking down the street. A cat is fighting the dog and a baby is crying. The baby is sleeping. The boy is playing on the swing. The man is laying down and the girl is jumping the jump rope. The lady is cooking chocolate chip cookies. A girl is going to the store. The man is going into the supermarket. The old man is fighting the other man. That's all. (Hedburg and Stoel-Gammon, 1986, p. 62)

Approximate age of emergence: 2 years

Sequences—Sequences represent the second stage of prenarrative development. The term *sequences* is confusing, since the elements of the stories are linked together by arbitrary commonalities but without a common characteristic. Sequence stories do include a macrostructure which involves a central character, topic, or setting. "The story elements are related to the central macrostructure on perceptual bonds" (Westby, 1984, p. 115). For example:

---

*Story examples adapted from *Topics in Language Disorders*, Vol. 7:1, pp. 62–64, with permission of Aspen Publishers, Inc., © December 1986.

Text reprinted from *Storybuilding: A Guide to Structuring Oral Narratives*, pp. 4–7, with permission of Thinking Publications, © 1990.

She lives with her dad. She lives with her mother. Grandma and Grandpa live together. And these three children live with their grandma. And these two animals live with them. And that's all. (Hedburg and Stoel-Gammon, 1986, p. 62)

Approximate age of emergence: 2 to 3 years

Primitive Narratives—Primitive narratives typify the next level of narrative development. Like the sequence stories, primitive narratives contain a macrostructure of a central character, topic, or setting. Unlike the sequences, the events in a primitive narrative follow from the central core. This main theme requires the child to interpret or predict events. "Children producing primitive narratives recognize and label facial expressions and body postures, and in their stories they make frequent reference to the associated feelings of the character" (Westby, 1984, p. 117). Children at this level of narrative development do not always recognize the reciprocal causality between thoughts and events (Larson and McKinley, 1987). Cohesive techniques such as use of pronominals and reiteration of the main character's name may be used. These techniques link individual sentences to the major theme but generally not to each other. For example:

My dad, he went up to go to work. My mom stayed and sleep in. My two brothers, they went to go play with the toys. My dog, she went outside. My kitty cat came up and he tickled me and came up and started to meow. And then I started to cry because he bit me. And my brothers came runnin' in and Mike said, "What happened?" They said, "What happened?" "My kitty cat just bit me." So mom comes runnin' in and she said, "What happened? Oh, the kitty cat bit you. O.K." (Hedburg and Stoel-Gammon, 1986, p. 62)

Approximate age of emergence: 3 to 4 years

Unfocused Chains—Unfocused chains are the next level of narrative development. These stories contain no central character or topic. Unfocused chains present an actual sequence of events yet there is no consistency of character or theme. The events are linked in logical or cause-effect relationships. Cohesive techniques of connecting words and propositions may appear. The conjunctions, *and, but,* and *because* may also be used. This type of narrative structure is seldom produced by children, for as soon as cause-effect and sequential relationships appear, children will begin to tie the story elements to each other and to a central theme (Westby, 1984). For example:

This man is walking. He saw a dog and a cat and he saw a girl, too, with the cat and the dog. He said, "Hello." He walked back and he said, "Brother, come here." So her grandmother walked up to her and said, "You wanna go dancing?" They went dancing. And so it was a slow dance. And then they went back. And then

258

these two children came. And then first he said, "I'm not." And then he said, "What?" "I wanna go out to eat." So they went out to eat. (Hedburg and Stoel-Gammon, 1986, p. 63)

Approximate age of emergence: 4 to 4½ years

Focused Chains—Focused chains are comprised of a central character with a logical sequence of events. These chains describe a chain of events that take the form of a series of "adventures." There are central characters and a true sequence of events but the listeners must interpret the ending. Westby (1984) states, "...the characters' actions seldom lead to attainment of a goal; consequently, if no goal is perceived, then, in the child's thinking, there is no need for an end to the story, or, at least, the ending does not have to follow logically from the beginning" (p. 118). For example:

> Once upon a time there was a mother named Christie. And she had a husband named Tom. And they had some children named Heather and Christie. And then they had a boy named Ronnie. And the mother told the boy to go outside to play. And then the boy came in and said, "Mother, mother, our dog's outside and he's barking. I will go see. What are you barking at? I don't know what he was barking at, Tommy, Ronnie, Ronnie. I don't know what he was barking at. You go out there and see. He wants in. I'll go let him in. There, I let him in." (Hedburg and Stoel-Gammon, 1986, p. 63)

Approximate age of emergence: 5 years

True Narratives—The level of true narratives represents the next stage of narrative development. True narratives adopt a consistent perspective focused on an incident in a story. There is a true plot, character development, and sequence of events. The presented problem, which is related to issues introduced in the beginning, is resolved in the end. Children may also perceive the relationship between attributes of characters and events. For example:

> One day there was a boy named Bobby and a girl named Sharon. They found a cat in their front yard and they brought it into the house. They fed the cat and they gave it some milk. They played and played with it and then a little while after a lady called and asked if anybody had seen her cat. And then they said that they had it at their house. And they brought it to the lady's house. And she gave them each five dollars for finding the cat and having them feed it and give it milk. (Hedburg and Stoel-Gammon, 1986, p. 64)

Approximate age of emergence: 6 to 7 years

Narrative Development After Seven Years of Age

Children's narrative development does not end at seven years of age. Rather, children seem to lengthen and refine their narratives. The elements of the narratives also grow more complex as the child matures (Applebee, 1978).

7–11 years of age—At this level of development, children will now begin to summarize and categorize stories. Children may categorize stories subjectively or objectively. "Subjectively, the child may categorize or summarize a story as 'funny' or 'exciting' or 'sad.' Objectively, the child may summarize a story as rhyming or long. In either case, the child is capable of considering the entire story and placing it in a more general category" (Larson and McKinley, 1987, p. 100).

11–12 years of age—Children at this level of development are now capable of producing complex stories with multiple embedded narrative structures.

13–15 years of age—Adolescents who reach this level of development are now adept at analyzing stories. This analysis is often combined with evaluation of stories or elements of stories.

16 years of age to adulthood—Individuals at this level of narrative development are now capable of more sophisticated analysis. When presented with a story, these individuals are now able to generalize about the story's meaning, formulate abstract statements about the message or theme of the story, and focus on their reaction to the story (Larson and McKinley, 1987).